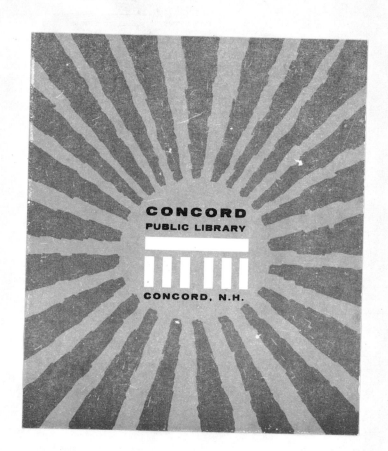

manya kahn body rhythms

manya kahn

body rhythms

a new approach to exercise

e. p. dutton

NEW YORK

Library of Congress Cataloging in Publication Data

Kahn, Manya.
   Body rhythms.

   1. Women—Health and hygiene. 2. Exercise for women. 3. Breathing exercises. I. Title.
RA778.K126   1977   613.7′04′5   76-52985

ISBN: 0-525-15275-X

Published simultaneously in Canada by Clarke, Irwin & Company Limited, Toronto and Vancouver

Edited by Pace Barnes
Designed by Betty Binns Graphics

All photographs by Charlotte Brooks, except pages 23–24 by Martin Bough

10 9 8 7 6 5 4 3 2 1

First Edition

To my grandchildren Ann, Peter, Jimmy, and Jean
and to all the loyal clients who encouraged me
to set my ideas down on paper

contents

you've got what it takes

Smart women today are enjoying a kind of personal freedom quite apart from political or social liberation. I call it "body freedom," and consider it not only every woman's inalienable right, but a responsibility she owes to herself. I'm talking about having a body that requires no binding girdles or uncomfortable waist cinchers to camouflage correctible imperfections. Every woman can develop a trim, youthful, flexible body naturally, and more and more are doing so now.

When I opened my first salon in New York City in 1941, beauty attitudes were very different; women believed that glamour and femininity were packaged assets to put on every morning and remove at night. Girdles in those days were regulation underdressing. Outward appearance was all most of them cared about, and it didn't have much to do with their real selves.

In the 1940s my clients were mostly middle-aged and wealthy. Exercise—save for the admittedly vain and pampered, or the orthopedically troubled—was very suspect. Women thought that exercise was drudgery or at the very least a bore. And the young believed either that youthful resiliency would last forever or that there was nothing you could do about the body's slowing down with age. But now . . . what a difference!

Today most women are ready to accept "new" ideas about exercise. These ideas only seem new because they formerly conflicted with mainstream thinking; actually they are the same ones I have always believed in and have used successfully to reshape women's bodies for thirty-five years! My clients now are both mature women and young, active women with both careers and families. They squeeze in time for exercise despite—and perhaps even because of—busy schedules. Today everyone is in search of a shapely body and an alert mind, both reflections of a capacity for living and of an enthusiasm for life.

how the manya kahn method evolved

This book is the expression of my philosophy derived from a life of working with thousands of women of all ages, first as a dancer and teacher of dance, then as a student of physical therapy, and now as a teacher of physical fitness. As a dancer, I marveled at the classic beauty and grace that could be developed through correct rhythmic body movement. I saw shy, awkward, and unattractive girls transformed as if by magic into exciting, beautiful women in an amazingly short time. Their new grace and beauty brought them new vitality, health, and joy in living.

Through the study of physical therapy, I learned of the wonders of the human body and how its abundant, natural resources, if well cared for, can preserve *youthful vitality for a lifetime.* I saw pitifully abused, sick bodies restored to normal health through correlated exercise, massage, corrective diet, and deep heat therapy, as well as hydrotherapy. I recognized how all these important natural factors, used so effectively in therapeutic work, could not only correct, but also prevent, the basic physical difficulties of women: overweight, underweight, impaired circulation, premature aging, nervous tension, and the inability to relax.

Body rhythms are based on natural, healthful measures When I opened my salon in 1941, I rejected the tiresome, enervating routines used in commercial salons and perfected a simple, *natural* method that healthfully revitalizes and rejuvenates the female body. I discarded all mechanical contrivances, starvation diets, and sweat methods because they are not only ineffective but drastically energy-depleting.

In order to strike at the roots of face and figure problems such as poor posture due to a weakened spinal column; soft, unused muscles notably in the abdomen, hips, and thighs; overindulgence in poorly balanced foods, I relied only on therapeutic measures—deep heat therapy, corrective Body Rhythms, and nutritional, well-balanced diets.

Some of my early clients, although delighted with the simplicity and ease of my methods, were skeptical at first. But after a few sessions, they were convinced my *natural* method was truly a health and beauty method that gave amazing results in a surprisingly short time.

I now have living proof that my theories were, and are, correct. Some of my clients, who came to me in their early forties, are still with me; they are now way past seventy. Their posture is perfect. Their bodies are free of aches and pains. They have no wrinkles in their faces. Their weight is ideal, and they look years younger than their actual ages.

It will take only ten days for you to discover an improvement in yourself, both in your looks and in your energy level. Following the 10-Day Health and Beauty Program correctly and at your own pace is all you need to adopt new and healthful habits that will last you for the rest of your life.

This book will show you how Body Rhythms work, in conjunction with proper breathing, relaxation, and diet, to develop your own potential for vitality and loveliness. There are continuing exercises beyond the 10-Day program for those who want to build greater physical flexibility and grace. Everyone's abilities and tolerances are different, just as everyone's needs are different. If you have a severe weight problem or a bad back, your needs are special but they are correctible.

how the manya kahn method differs from all others

Over the last 35 years I have seen the most appalling crash diets, endless gadgets, reducing machines, and all sorts of exercise fads come and go. During the last few years, however, I have seen the approach to exercise and diet become more realistic despite continuing fads.

In my system for body conditioning I have never used energy-depleting gymnastics—aimless fast-moving, jerky routines. These movements are performed at the expense of the energy and vitality that all of us are trying to develop in the first place! These tiring exercises do nothing but add bulk by hardening muscle and fatty tissue, as well as bring on tension and fatigue. They should be banished forever!

Artificial dehydration is another method of which I never approved. I'm talking about enervating sweat cabinets, steam rooms, and sauna baths that have become popular because of their false promise of immediate weight loss.

So-called reducing equipment such as weighted belts and vibrating belts, stationary bicycles, vibrating tables, and all other mechanical contraptions too numerous to mention are more props I rejected. These debilitating gadgets cannot possibly help you lose weight. The only things you really lose are time, energy and vitality!

I have also discarded all crash and starvation diets that leave the face tired-looking and gaunt, the muscle tissue of the body soft and flabby. These destructive measures ruin a woman's appearance and lessen energy and vitality. Down goes the spirit as well!

you're never too young or too old

When you are in your teens   In the formative, adolescent years, you are cutting the pattern for the person you will be at thirty, at forty, and for the rest of your life. If you know some simple facts about the importance of the spinal column, of why muscles must be exercised properly to maintain the natural corseting of the body, of what a properly balanced diet can mean in the way of acquiring a clear skin, hair with natural sheen, and all the elements that make for attractiveness—then your way through the years is cleared.

When you are in your twenties   The twenties are the years that will mold the shape of your body, your attitudes and your ways of thinking. No longer is an exuberant awkwardness tolerated because of your youth. Draping yourself in a slouch is inexcusable. As time goes on, your body will protest in the forms of a weakened back, a protruding abdomen and posterior, a drooping chin, possibly dowager's hump at the back of your neck, and, most certainly, nagging fatigue. If you follow the plan of this book, you can build something quite different from this doleful picture of your future.

Should you fall into the category of a "plain" girl, I assure you that with intelligent effort and self-discipline, your awkward body can be molded into good lines, pleasantly proportioned in inches and pounds, and can be trained to move with grace. Poor skin will become clearer and finer-textured, merely through diet and more sensible living habits. An unwieldy body will respond to muscle discipline with good posture and grace of movement. A dour disposition will become happy and responsive as a result

8

of a sense of well-being. Deliberately achieved, these attributes have a more powerful effect over oneself and others than does shallow prettiness. That is why the "plain" girl so often becomes the woman of true feminine charm, grace, and dignity.

The thirties are full of exciting possibilities! In her thirties, a woman has perspective. She has begun to realize that everyone has troubles, and she learns to handle disappointments with philosophical good humor. She is at her peak mentally and physically. Never before has she been so charming, so intelligent, so well balanced. Yet there are many women who allow themselves to become overworked, overtired, and tense. Instead of developing a relaxed attitude toward life, they nag and tear at it. They demand perfection of themselves, their families, and their children. The added burdens create tension which can be a distressing, disrupting factor. The answer is in discovering the art of relaxation.

If you do not know how to relax, learn. The thirties fly by like no other years. If you neglect yourself physically, you can become truly middle-aged before your time. If you remain healthy and physically attractive, the mind and spirit invariably follow, and you will welcome the forties with both the appearance and spirit of youth, and with poise and confidence.

Forty with a new-found freedom! The forties bring a new freedom to every healthy woman. For the first time books are being written with titles like "The Wonderful Crisis of Middle Age." It is a time when responsibilities like childbearing are over. One knows oneself; emotions are more stable and enjoyment is keen and sharp. If you have neglected yourself and allowed the marks of age to creep in, you may think that the weary droop of your shoulders, the squarishness of your figure, and the heavy feeling in your legs and feet are things that will be with you forever. Don't believe it for a minute. You can rediscover your lovely, lithe, youthful self once again, in spite of the fears of approaching menopause.

Menopause This once-dreaded time is a perfectly natural occurrence. It is no mystery and it is no longer feared. The reproductive function ceases and your childbearing time is past. Although bodily readjustments must take place and certain physi-

cal reactions may or may not manifest themselves, your condition of health is largely responsible for the extent of your discomfort during this period. When your health is good, when you know you can take pride in your looks, you may be all but unconscious of this cyclic change, and life can continue to be full and rich.

Conversely, a woman in poor health may find this a trying period in her life. She is apt to carry around a "sorry for herself" attitude. As a result, she shuts out all the fine and good things in her life, and discouraging attitudes gain ground. The general symptoms are nervousness and tension. At this time, it is more important than ever to learn to let tension and strain go. Learn to relax by applying my general health principles. By combating the minor and exaggerated physical disturbances and moods of this period you will have taken a giant step toward health, beauty, and personal charm. Remember that the ending of the menstrual period is just as natural as the beginning, and that its trials, like all things, pass with time. Life can be even better afterward!

The general misconception that a woman's feminine appeal is terminated after menopause is not only untrue but absurd. Nothing is further from the truth. The natural bodily adjustments will have no disagreeable effect on the woman who is healthy and attractive—on the contrary! When fears of pregnancy are gone we are usually more relaxed, and relaxation is the precious ingredient in everyone's sex life. Time and again I have been told by my clients that their sexual activities actually increased and proved to be much more enjoyable. I assure you life can be even better than before.

The mature, rewarding years—the fifties, sixties and seventies! Women who have kept good health and retained attractiveness into maturity are as a rule the happiest. If you are beginning to show signs of age and are conscious of aches and pains, stiffness in body movement, a lack of enjoyment in walking because of your general physical discomforts, this is the time to say, "I shall not grow old indifferently." Though you may find it takes time and patience to undo the results of careless living—I assure you it can be done, provided you are not actually ill. You can, with my commonsense program, gradually bring back the health and good looks that are rightfully yours regardless of your years. The Body Rhythm method is gentle, gradual, and in no

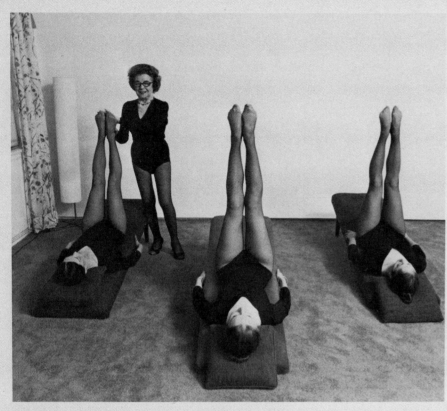

Manya Kahn instructs at her salon in New York City.

sense strenuous, and follows natural principles for promoting good health. It substitutes knowledge and control for ignorance and lack of control. What is true for the fifties is also true of the sixties and seventies. Stiffness and old-age mannerisms can be phased out and replaced by an ageless and classical charm that is appropriate for your age. And you can enjoy the maturing years with grace and good humor.

Intelligent understanding is vital in performing any job well and certainly most essential before starting on a physical fitness program. The following pages in this book will give you that understanding and, hopefully, the inspiration and determination to follow through. Conflicting notions about the human body still exist, but you can replace conjecture with knowledge if you follow and absorb what you learn. Your health and the natural beauty that comes with it are your heritage. It is your responsibility to nurture that heritage toward glowing good health and good looks.

It is my hope that you will take this book very seriously. It is a program for many years to come; it will always remind you that health is your most precious possession. Good health is what makes your appearance vital and attractive and your mind alert, hopeful and resourceful, ever ready to accept change as it is mirrored in the ever-new, day-by-day experiences. Good health is our one assault-proof armor in this age of high tempo and tense living.

manya kahn body rhythms

manya kahn
body rhythms
—a new approach
to exercise

the natural way to health and beauty

Nature has endowed the human body with an amazing abundance of vital resources to preserve health and youthful vitality through a lifetime. But women today often ignore these natural potentialities for staying young and attractive. In their frantic desire for a lovelier face and a shapelier body, they resort to energy-depleting, often dangerous diets, to excessive dehydration, and strenuous routines of exercise, with results that are not only temporary and illusory, but injurious and destructive as well.

What good is a loss of weight if, as a result, your face is tired-looking and gaunt? What good is a trim figure if you lack animation and energy? What good is a drastically dieted body that is lost in fat as soon as you return to normal eating habits?

There are no miracle shortcuts to health and beauty. Emphasis must be placed on building basic good health, sensibly and consistently. For only then can we develop and attain long-lasting health, youthful vitality, and natural beauty.

The only intelligent and permanent way to achieve the good looks we envy in others who obviously take care of themselves is to follow a regular, scientifically planned program of physical activity that will firm muscle tone, redistribute weight evenly, and strengthen the entire muscle structure of the body.

Now that women of all ages have changed their attitudes about exercise, such a regime is both acceptable and possible. Women want to feel alive and look attractive and they have learned from experimenting with other methods that good health and good looks cannot be achieved through starvation diets, reducing machines, magic lotions, or beauty creams.

To replace old-fashioned methods of exercise, I have created a unique system of corrective, rhythmic, almost effortless body movements I call "Body Rhythms." These Body Rhythms, which are proven to be anatomically and functionally correct, are performed in a slow stretch/breathe/relax sequence coordinated with deep breathing. These movements have time and again shown themselves effective in correcting specific face and figure problems, such as premature aging, overweight, sluggish circulation, underweight, bad posture, tension, and fatigue.

I have successfully used this system to reshape the bodies of both young and older women alike. The routines must be practiced consistently to make up for any lack of regular muscular activity, which may have resulted—if we have let it—in a gradual slowdown and deterioration of all our body functions, not to mention the energy and spirits that tend to sag along with the flesh.

A great majority of women and men feel exhausted much of the time and blame this condition either on overexertion or the stresses of our frantic, contemporary style of living. This is a comfort for the passive and pessimistic among us who prefer to give in, but it is a false comfort. In my opinion it is not normal to feel listless or fatigued all the time at any age.

We got ourselves into this predicament because the shortcuts of contemporary life limit the free function and movement of the body's entire muscle structure. Many of us go through life with an apathetic minimum of movement. Where we used to carry, lift, walk, and run, we now press buttons and wait. Our jobs require the limited use of only a few muscles, and even when we golf, ski, or play tennis we do not use all the muscles of the body, and the few we do use we overexert. The result is that we are at once tired and flabby, an uncomfortable state of being.

But there is someone else we can blame partly for our discomfort: our ancestors, because they refused to walk on all fours and instead assumed an upright position. We take it for granted that this is the way it was meant to be, but the upright position actually puts too much strain on the body's major support area, the lumbar region of the spine. It is this strain that is the source of so many of our complaints—general fatigue, tension, and backaches, more common now than the common cold. But these are not problems we should be prepared to live with. We can counteract and even overcome them through the development of good posture; and that begins with strengthening those flabby, unused muscles!

getting down to basics

Figure faults in women are often due to unused muscles in the diaphragm, abdomen, waist, hips, and thighs, which express their uselessness and strain by collapsing. This results in the creation of that dismal spread that young women anticipate with dread, and that middle-aged women lament. But inactive muscles do much more damage; they also slow up the circulation of the blood, causing fatigue and general lassitude. Since more than half of the body's weight consists of muscle tissue, we can easily understand why habitual lack of corrective body movements slows all the bodily functions and the circulation as well.

Muscles in action stretch, contract, and relax. The blood vessels follow suit by stretching, contracting, and relaxing in turn. When the bloodstream is stimulated and quickened through proper body movements, good circulation is created and is then able to feed the entire body more efficiently. When muscular activity is correct, it also creates pulsations and contractions in the tissues known and defined as muscle tone. Firm muscle tone creates a feeling of being alive, of having the strength and ability to perform physical tasks for long periods of time without tiring. Good muscle tone gives firmness and slender lines to the body and is the basis for good health and good posture.

The most effective way of stimulating circulation and developing good muscle tone is to learn the correct movements for all body muscles. Body Rhythms are designed to teach you these movements, in order to help you shape, mold, strengthen, and firm all flabby and weak areas in the body. Special emphasis is placed on the muscles of the diaphragm, abdomen, buttocks, hips, and thighs, for it is the muscles of these areas on which the whole body, including the spine, depends for its major support. Good posture, the fundamental and too often ignored source of health and beauty, can never be attained through mere admonitions, familiar to all of us, to "Stand Up Straight." We cannot stand up straight unless the important muscles that support the spine and entire body structure are in perfect condition.

I cannot overemphasize the fact that the muscles of the body must be brought back into activity. The question you might ask is

"How? Wouldn't any form of exercise do?" My answer is "Definitely Not!" and you will easily understand why when the concept of Body Rhythms is explained in detail.

the three major principles of body rhythms

There are three major principles upon which I built the entire system of Body Rhythms. The first is based on a slow stretch/breathe/relax technique which consists of stretching the body thoroughly, breathing deeply, and relaxing completely with each movement.

The second principle is based on the rhythmic movements a child follows in its progressive stages of natural physical development from infancy to maturity.

We all know that a newborn baby lies flat on its back and is unable to lift the body to a sitting position. The reason is obvious: the spine is not strong enough, nor are the muscles. When we try to prop the baby up, the head droops, because the spinal column is underdeveloped and weak. However, nature has provided the human race with wonderful instincts for growth and physical development.

Prone position During the first months, while in a prone position, the baby instinctively gains strength in the muscles by moving constantly. It stretches the body, yawning frequently to take in large quantities of oxygen, and continually moves the arms and legs. All these natural movements strengthen the muscles of the chest, abdomen, hips, thighs, and lower back, developing its body, thus preparing it for the next stage of growth.

Sitting up In the sitting position further development takes place, primarily in the dorsal region. The baby instinctively moves from the hip joints forward and sideways, and stretches upward. The upward arm movements strengthen the chest, upper shoulders, and diaphragm. And, again, all these movements prepare the baby for the next important step.

Crawling It is in the crawling stage that the spinal column is developed and strengthened. The supportive muscles also gain strength, as do the arms and legs. When this is accomplished, the child is ready for the major and final stage of physical development—the attainment of erect posture.

Standing From an upright position the child continues to exercise the body to develop sufficient stamina for walking and finally for running.

As you begin the basic program you will discover that the Body Rhythms routines follow the identical movements of a child's natural physical development from infancy to full growth. Executed in five different positions—lying down, sitting, half-reclining, kneeling, and standing, this system has worked wonders in retraining, strengthening, and reshaping the adult female body to graceful, feminine proportions.

The third principle concentrates on developing and strengthening the spinal column to enable it to provide the necessary support to the entire body. The section that follows will enlighten you on the major role the spinal column plays in the anatomy of the human body and how crucial it is to counteract the inherent weaknesses of the spine.

The complete Body Rhythms program is divided into three groups: Basic or Elementary, Intermediate, and Advanced. The purpose of this breakdown is to enable you to re-educate and revitalize all the weak muscles in the body gradually without strain, without tension, and without fatigue. The basic routines must be perfected before the intermediate group is attempted. The advanced routines should follow only after the first and second groups have been accomplished. This is the only intelligent, efficient, and successful method to help you achieve desirable results and to enable you to put your body into perfect physical condition for many years to come.

Once you develop the habit of practicing Body Rhythms regularly, you will want to incorporate them into a regular and continuing daily schedule of activities. They will become an integral part of your new, healthful, and exciting way of life.

the spinal column
— the life line of
the body

One of the most important things to understand about my system of Body Rhythms is that it is based on my conviction that the spinal column is *the life line of our body structure,* upon which our mental and physical state of well-being depends. The stronger the backbone, the firmer the muscle tone surrounding the lower back, and the more perfectly the spinal column is aligned, the healthier we are. Therefore, we are more able to function normally and efficiently in all our daily activities, whether we work, swim, play tennis, golf, ski, dance, or walk.

A weak and underdeveloped spine creates *bad posture* and the entire body acts like a "broken-down machine" ready to fall apart. All the important parts of the body, bones, muscles, joints, nerves, and all vital organs, are cramped into inactivity and become sluggish and practically lifeless. Is there any wonder that backaches are so prevalent?

Conversely, a healthy, strong and well-developed spine creates *good posture* and makes one feel alive, alert, full of energy and youthful vitality. Because the spinal column is so instrumental in the achievement of good health and perfect posture, it is important that you understand first its basic structure before I discuss the inherent weaknesses that cause back problems.

the intricate structure of the spine

The spine consists of twenty-four small bones called vertebrae, which, for descriptive purposes, can be divided into five groups. The first seven, or cervical vertebrae are at the back of the neck and extend downward from the head. The topmost of these, the atlas, is the smallest of the vertebrae, and its function is to support the head. The second cervical bone, or the axis, forms a pivot for the first vertebra upon which the head can rotate. The remaining five are called simply cervicals.

The next group of twelve vertebrae are the thoracic group; they form the trunk and have accompanying ribs. These vertebrae increase in size from the upper back downward and encompass the area housing the lungs, heart, liver, and stomach.

Below the thoracic are the five lumbar vertebrae, which lie directly behind the abdomen and form what we call the "small" of the back. They serve as attachments for the pelvis and are linked with the abdominal organs. These are the largest and strongest vertebrae in the movable part of the spinal column. Their extra length, thickness, and width give the greatest support to the body as a whole.

The fourth group consists of five sacral vertebrae. They are part of the pelvis, protecting the female organs and the lower intestines. In early life they consist of five separate bones, but these bones gradually grow together with age, forming a triangle in the lower part of the spinal column called the sacrum. This sacrum acts as a wedge between the two hip bones. The last five vertebrae at the lowest end of the spine also fuse with time and form a triangular group called the coccyx.

Each vertebra, from the tiniest at the very top of the spine to the largest at the very bottom of the lumbar region, forms a ring through which the spinal cord is threaded. This constitutes the important link between mental and physical well-being.

The complete spine has about 1,000 ligaments (very strong tissues) which attach one bone to another. There are also a great number of tendons which attach the muscles to the bones. In addition, there are about 150 small joints. The joints singly permit only slight movement but together give enough elasticity to the spinal column to allow us to bend and stretch in all directions: forward, backward, and sideways. Cushioning each joint is a light elastic tissue called cartilage. Through constant stretching and movement of the spine, this cartilage cushion thickens, enabling us to move with great ease and without conscious effort.

A perfectly aligned spinal column gives the body the necessary support for good posture. Any deviation from a perfect alignment of the spine, whether minor, acute, or chronic, is the major cause of back problems. The question now is what to do to correct already existing difficulties and how to prevent them in the future.

the bad back syndrome

Recent statistics tell us there are literally millions of people who suffer from bad back problems. This proves that nature has endowed the human race with a weak and underdeveloped spinal column. Therefore, to develop a strong, healthy back is something most of us have to work for to attain. The sooner we acknowledge this fact the sooner we will be able to correct it.

So that you can understand the bad back syndrome more thoroughly, it is essential that we learn its origin and its causes. To comprehend the evolution of human locomotion and its relation to good posture, it is important to put this whole subject into proper perspective. The following information should do just that.

The evolution of human locomotion The human body is admirably engineered to perform a wide variety of functions. Unfortunately, *walking upright* is not one of them. Our ancestors, from whom we inherit our basic body structure, moved about by swinging through the trees; if they had to get about on the ground at all, they did so on all fours. They had long powerful shoulders and arms, and they used their thighs, legs, and feet for reaching, holding, gripping but only rarely for standing on.

When our ancestors finally took to the ground they walked at first rather like gorillas or chimpanzees, bent forward at the hip joints with the weight of the upper body supported by their powerful arms and knuckles. The tilt of the pelvis of the most recent human ancestor, who was still more ape than man, indicates he walked on flat feet tilting forward from the hip joints and moved on all fours when real speed was required. Therefore, his stance for moving on the ground was the first adaptation of the original structural body design for tree swinging.

The first human ancestor considered *true man* is called Homo Erectus, specifically because the most significant adaptation he made was to walk entirely *upright*. Erect posture is thus a second adaptation of human locomotion. It required that the entire weight of the upper body be supported by the spinal column and especially by the lower back, which was originally a fragile pivot as compared to the powerful shoulders, arms, and legs. The legacy of this adoption is strain on some muscles, under use of others, and—you guessed it—back trouble. *Nature evidently never intended the back to be a support column.*

Sitting down is a third adaptation, in addition to standing upright and walking on all fours. Sitting at great length is the major culprit of our *sedentary* way of life. Sitting at a desk for hours, watching television for hours, sitting in the movies for long periods of time, reading for hours in a badly postured chair—all not only create a terrific strain in the lower back, but also aggravate the existing problems caused by the upright position. But since sitting and standing are unavoidable in our civilized way of life, it is imperative that we immediately embark on a necessary program to correct and prevent back problems. This exercise program must be based on a system that is anatomically and functionally correct, geared specifically to strengthen and revitalize the spine.

This brings us to the subject of *exercise*. Most orthopedic doctors today agree that the only salvation for the millions of sufferers with back pains is exercise, but not the conventional or ordinary kind. I am talking about gymnastics or calisthenics, the kind we are all taught to do in gym class. In school we are drilled to do push-ups, sit-ups, knee bends, toe touching, performed fast and jerky at the expense of energy and vitality. We have all experienced the painful results of this form of exercise: sore muscles, more tension, and greater fatigue. Often more serious and injurious side effects take place, such as acute backaches, often even hernias, and in more extreme cases—heart attacks.

For years we have been conditioned to believe this is the only way to keep fit. The sad fact is that this harmful system is still practiced in schools and in commercial gyms throughout the country where women and men seek help to improve their physical condition and outward appearance. But most of the time their efforts are in vain, which I think is deplorable and unfortunate.

To replace existing and undesirable systems of exercise, I evolved an entirely new method of movement called Body Rhythms. Relying on this method for thirty-five years and judging by the wonderful results acheived by my clients who were referred to me by their physicians, I am convinced Body Rhythms are most effective in ridding the body of the various back problems that make life miserable.

Pregnancy may also cause problems of the spine Pregnant women who never exercised in their childhood or adolescent years often develop back pains during pregnancy and even after childbirth. The cause, naturally, is poorly developed abdominal muscles and a weak spinal column due to muscular inactivity. The enlarged protrusion in the abdomen often causes an exaggerated swayback which puts a terrific strain on posture and is one more cause of stress and discomfort in the lumbar region.

In my experience, however, those pregnant women who, in their younger years, appreciated the value of exercise and engaged in all sorts of athletic activities never exhibited any painful reactions despite their pregnancies. Their well-developed spinal column were strong enough and able to adjust to the stress and strain that pregnancy usually inflicts.

The pregnant women referred to me by their gynecologists who continued to practice Body Rhythms throughout the nine months were also free of all pains and aches and had remarkably easy childbirths. Their postnatal recoveries came about quickly and with the greatest of ease. It is gratifying to know that these days doctors advise their women patients to exercise not only during pregnancy, but also before and after.

Mental upsets—another major cause of back problems Until now I have only discussed the physical problems of weak and ailing backs. There is, however, another major cause— mental stress and emotional upheavals which invariably cause strain, tension, and prolonged fatigue. These symptoms often lead to contractions and spasms in the muscle tissue surrounding the back and can inflict real pain and discomfort despite the fact there are no physical complications.

In mild cases the cure may come about by simply learning how to relax (see section on relaxation). The more serious and acute cases, however, are definitely in the realm of a psychiatrist. The most aggravated cases are the ones which, in addition to mental upsets, are also inflicted with physical difficulties. The treatment of both problems should be undertaken simultaneously by specialists in their respective fields as quickly as possible.

Whether your particular problem was diagnosed by your physician as sciatica, lumbago, slipped disc or by any other name, I assure you that all these difficulties are due primarily to the weakness of the spine caused by physical inactivity and its continued lack of proper treatment. As we grow older these problems become more acute, often chronic, and it takes much longer to eliminate them. Since eliminate them we must, there is no other way to succeed but to start to *exercise promptly and correctly.*

body rhythms will correct and cure back problems

By now you should be as enlightened as I am about the origin and cause of our back ailments and resolve to eliminate them or to prevent them. To succeed you must embark immediately on the program of Body Rhythms illustrated on pages 19–21 It is a short program specially designed for women who suffer from back ailments.

Before you start on the special 10-Day Program, you must first concentrate on the preliminary Body Rhythms until your back is cured of all aches and pains. By practicing daily as instructed, these corrective movements will, no doubt, heal existing problems and hopefully prevent a recurrence in the future. Before you start, however, you will be wise to consult your personal physician, who is, after all, the best judge of your back problem.

Chronic back ailments ruin health, disposition and the ability to perform our daily responsibilities efficiently. So start practicing immediately and you will soon note a great improvement in your strength, stamina and appearance.

It is my hope that you read this chapter with great interest. The newly acquired knowledge should encourage you to include Body Rhythms in your daily schedule. For only then will you succeed in erasing the bad back syndrome. A life free of pains and aches can be a joyous and delightful experience.

body rhythm I

FULL BODY STRETCH

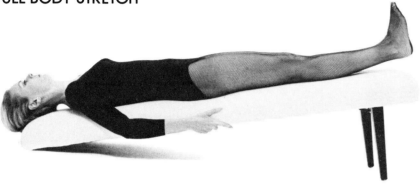

STARTING POSITION

Lie flat on slantboard with lower part of back touching board, knees straight, arms at sides, hands grasping board, toes pointed.

From Starting Position, flex both feet, bringing toes toward you, pushing heels out to straighten knees.

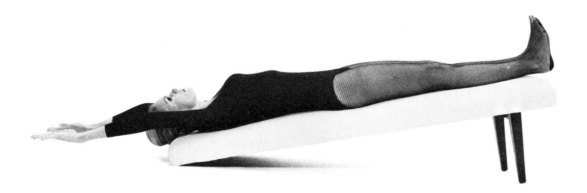

Breathe in while you stretch both arms out sideways, then back, stretching elbows and fingers at the same time. Hold for one second.

Breathe out while returning slowly to Starting Position. Relax.

Repeat five times.

body rhythms

for back ailments

Body rhythms I-V are corrective movements to activate the spinal column, pelvic area, and abdominal region. They are performed with double legs only. Single leg movements stretch the spine unevenly and can cause further pain and injury.

These preliminary Body Rhythms should be practiced daily until your back is free of aches and pains and you can begin the 10-Day Program. For greater results, work on a slantboard.

Remember to work with slow, sustained, rhythmic motions coordinated with deep breathing. Never strain.

If you have a **chronic** back problem, you must consult your physician before attempting the Body Rhythms program.

body rhythm II

DOUBLE LEG STRETCH

From Starting Position, flex both feet, keeping knees straight (a).

Breathe in and bring both legs straight up to vertical position. Bounce back and forth three times from hip joints (b).

Breathe out as both legs are slowly lowered to Starting Position. Relax.

Repeat five times.

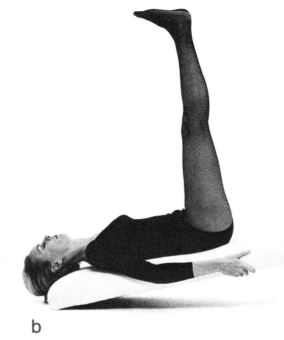

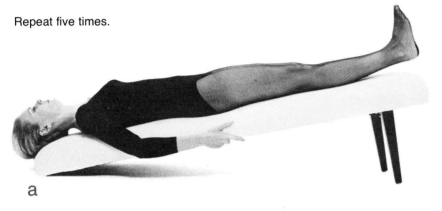

a

b

body rhythm III

DOUBLE KNEE STRETCH

From Starting Position, **breathe in**, bend both knees (c), placing feet flat on slantboard.

Breathe out, bring both knees into chest. Bounce knees back and forth toward chest three times from hip joints (d).

Breathe in, stretch both legs straight up with toes pointed, knees straight (b). Flex both feet, bring both legs slowly down as you **breathe out.** Relax.

Repeat five times.

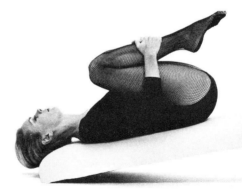

d

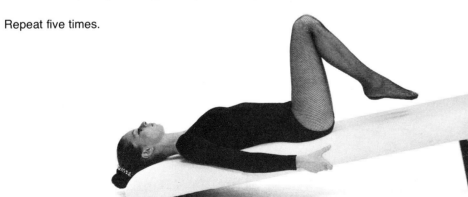

c

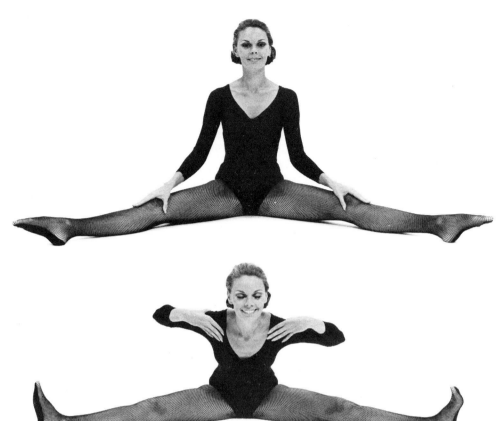

body rhythm V

TORSO STRETCH

STARTING POSITION

Stand erect with feet pointing forward about 10 inches apart, arms at sides, elbows straight.

From Starting Position, clasp hands behind you, keeping elbows straight.

Breathe in, stretch arms back and up as far as possible with head going up at same time. Hold for three seconds. **Breathe out.** Relax.

Breathe in. Bend torso forward, moving from hip joints. Stretch arms way up simultaneously. Be sure back is straight, abdomen pulled in.

Breathe out. Bounce 3 times from hip joints.

Breathe in. Return to upright position. **Breathe out.**

Repeat five times.

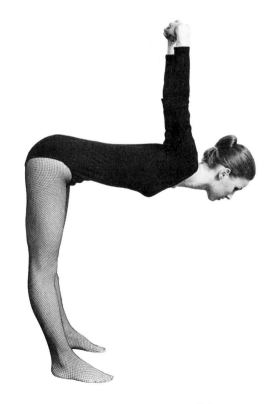
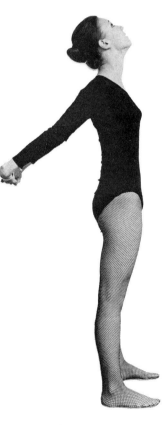

body rhythm IV

TORSO BENDS

STARTING POSITION

Sit on floor, spine as straight as possible, shoulders relaxed, abdomen pulled in, legs stretched wide apart, knees straight.

From Starting Position, **breathe in** as you place both palms on shoulders, raise elbows straight out to shoulder level with back straight.

Flex feet. **Breathe out**, moving from hip joints, stretch torso forward and down as far as possible. Bounce up and down from hip joints three times.

Breathe in, return to center. **Breathe out.**

Repeat five times.

good posture
— the foundation of
health and beauty

Have you ever seen a truly beautiful woman enter a crowded room? All eyes turn to her because she glides in gracefully, bringing with her a certain aura of elegance, a special glow. Invariably she carries herself erectly, with great self-assurance and grace. It is this erectness and grace that makes the difference between simple good looks and breathtaking loveliness. Straight shoulders—a proud uplift of the head, neck, and chest—ease of motion and grace of bearing—these are the qualities that set the beautiful woman apart.

Good posture and carriage are fundamental sources of glowing good health, real glamour, and beauty. Moreover, the way you stand, walk, and carry yourself lets the world know exactly what you think of yourself. It often determines what others think of you as well.

The dictionary defines posture as an "attitude," which can mean both mental and physical. Never separate the two! Your attitude toward yourself and toward life in general is reflected just as much in the way you sit, stand, and walk as it is in how you act and what you say. When you slouch, your body is pulled downward by the force of gravity—hardly the picture of buoyant self-confidence!

We hear a great deal these days about the proper way to sit, stand, and walk to achieve good posture. Some say, "Press the small of your back against the wall." Others say, "Pull in your abdomen," "tuck in your buttocks." But all these well-meaning suggestions are superficial remedies that never really succeed in developing good posture.

How, then, can you achieve good posture? First, you must learn how to develop a strong and elastic spine, one that will give proper support to the body in an upright position and allow free movement and stretching in all directions.

To succeed, you need to follow a program of corrective body movements that will strengthen and firm the large muscles of the body, mainly those in the diaphragm, abdomen, hips, buttocks, and thighs. These muscles must be strong, firm, and well-developed to give proper support to the entire weight of the body. Body Rhythms 1 through 6 will do just that if followed correctly and faithfully! These movements are the very cornerstones upon which good posture can be built.

The importance of the spine in the achievement of good posture cannot be overemphasized. The spinal column is, after all, the major support for all the organs of the body, and a unifying link among them. It is also closely related to the nervous system. Proper care of the spinal region, in order for it to perform its vital functions with natural ease and without hindrance of any kind, is therefore crucial, and an awareness of the spine's contribution to general good health and good posture is essential to that care.

Dowager's hump, rounded shoulders, and other atrocities of poor posture Poor posture, if prolonged, can mold bone and muscle into a permanent pattern and cause deformation of the spinal column. The major symptoms are dowager's hump, rounded shoulders, sunken chest, lateral curvature (known as scoliosis), and, in the lumbar region, swayback, also known as lordosis. These common posture faults are deplorable signs of old age which, too often, are even seen on young women.

Women develop these posture habits in different ways. For the most part, habits form unconsciously. Some women slouch while reading, sewing, or sitting at a desk. Others droop physically when they become tired, worried, or depressed. A great many rest by slouching in soft chairs. As the cycle of bad habits continues, nervousness, tenseness, and exhaustion increase.

Watch out for girdles and high-heeled shoes! Modern attire also helps to further the cause of poor posture. The tight girdle is a real culprit, as it greatly restricts free movement. High heels are another menace. They throw the body off balance and put severe strain on the spine whenever the wearer walks or stands. Too much weight is shifted to the metatarsal arch of the foot, instead of being distributed evenly. The pelvis is tilted and the abdomen thrown forward. The answer to all these problems is to change from high to low heels as frequently as possible. As for tight girdles, do not resort to them! They encourage sluggish circulation and add to the weakness and flabbiness in the major muscles in the body. A neat appearance can be achieved with a light, two-way-stretch garment. Once you reshape your body with Body Rhythms, you'll have no need to wear one!

guidelines for standing, sitting, walking tall

To improve posture you need no special equipment except your own body and a determination to succeed. A full-length mirror is helpful for analyzing your problems. When you have strengthened the large muscles of your body through Body Rhythms, you'll find it much easier to stand tall, sit tall, and think tall. Both your abdominal and derrière problems will be corrected also. Once you gain control over your lower back area, your abdominal muscles will automatically pull in and flatten out, and your buttocks will fall into proper line. These strengthened areas will gradually begin to respond to better posture. The new posture habits may feel strange at first, so it is important to concentrate and make sure you retain them.

When you have assumed the proper, erect, easy carriage, you will marvel at the difference it makes in excess pounds and inches if you are overweight. If you are too thin, the proper alignment of your body—with shoulders pulled back and chest out—can add inches to your bust and pounds to other parts of your body. When your body functions properly, it works like a precise machine, smoothly and effortlessly. With all parts in proper alignment, the head is held high, neck and shoulders are relaxed, and the abdomen is firm and flat enough to form its own natural corset. Your arms and legs assume their natural position, and rhythmic, graceful movement comes automatically.

Sitting As you probably have noticed, sitting down is something few people manage to do with much grace. Actually,

Illustrated below are correct positions for working at a table or desk.

When reading, use a straight chair and sit with torso as far back as possible, shoulders and back straight, chest out, abdomen pulled in; keep knees and feet together. Books or other reading matter should be propped up. This angle is healthier for the eyes and will prevent dropping of the head, causing dowager's hump.

Read no more than one hour at a time, then get up and move about to awaken circulation.

For writing (or dining), sit back as shown and move torso forward from the hip joints. Keep the back straight, chest out, abdomen in. This will stretch the lower back and avoid shoulder strain.

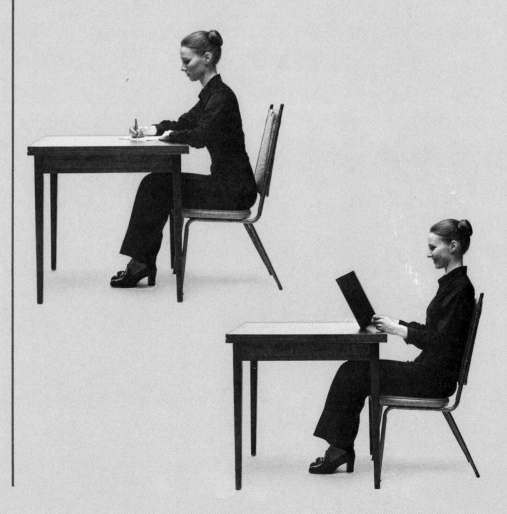

When picking up objects, people normally bend their torsos forward stretching from the shoulders instead of moving from the hip joints. Leading with the shoulders strains and rounds out the upper part of the back creating bad posture.

Instead assume a squat position by bending the knees and lowering the torso level with the knees, spine straight, shoulders relaxed, head up.

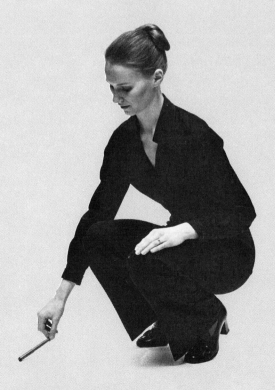

it is not difficult at all. The three main points to remember are to sit tall, sit way back in the seat of the chair, and sit on your pelvic bones, not on your spine; your arms and hands should be relaxed, resting on your lap or on the arms of the chair. Your legs should also be relaxed, with your feet fairly close together. If you must cross your legs, cross them at the ankles and nowhere else! You may not realize it, but it makes them look bigger. In general, the more correctly you sit, the longer you can sit comfortably. That will be a good thing to remember the next time you start to squirm at a movie theater!

Lowering yourself onto a couch or chair is another everyday movement that you may need to work on. Don't "plunk" your body down as if it were a bundle of falling packages. This looks terrible! It also makes you look old and awkward. Instead, stand against the chair with one foot slightly ahead of the other to help balance your body. Now tuck your buttocks under, hold the upper part of your body erect, and, keeping your knees slightly bent, lower yourself slowly into the chair. All of this, of course, should be done as one fluid movement.

To get up, draw your feet in slightly, then put one foot ahead of the other. With the ball of the back foot as close to the chair as possible, lean forward from the hips. Keeping your back straight, lift yourself up from the chair. Be sure you don't use your arms as a lever. If you are short, try to sit in a chair that will accommodate you—one with shorter legs. If one is not available, it is best to sit on the edge of your seat with your feet touching the floor.

Bending forward and walking The proper way to bend forward when you're standing or sitting is from the hip joints, and with an absolutely straight back, rather than from the shoulders, which is what most people do. When you move the torso forward from the shoulders, posture is ruined. But when you bend forward from the hip joints, the lower back begins to stretch, which helps the knees to relax tension and rigidity.

Correct posture is also the basis for walking correctly, with head up, shoulders back, abdomen in, buttocks under, knees straight. Here's the way to do it: With the weight of your body on the outside of your feet, point your toes straight ahead and try to keep as close as possible to a single imaginary line.

Make your strides by swinging forward from the hip joints,

not from the knees. When you do this, your stride will be longer. Avoid mincing steps. Try breathing deeply as you walk, to help your stride and rhythm. Be sure you don't drag or shuffle your feet; lift them off the ground for each step. Remember that the heel goes down first, the ball of the foot next. Walk lightly at all times without swinging your hips or your arms. And as you walk, contract your buttock muscles to prevent swaying.

When you go up a staircase, keep your back straight and head up. Let your thighs do the work. With one foot on the step above, lift your chest and move up. When you descend, bend the forward knee deeply and place your toes on the lower step. Transfer your weight to the other foot and repeat the movement. Don't watch your foot. Keep your eyes straight ahead instead. This is a real tip-off to your degree of self-confidence!

general hints for good posture

1. To apply your good posture habits to routine chores, remember the principles of proper alignment.

2. When you lift a heavy object, let your thighs and legs bear most of the burden. Don't reach for the object while in a standing position. Instead, lower your body, flexing your knees. As you raise the object, push up with your thighs to an upright position.

3. It is better to carry two evenly divided bundles in both hands than one large bundle in one hand. This avoids straining the shoulders.

4. If you must carry a heavy load each day, like books, alternate the arm in which you carry them in order to balance and redistribute the constant weight.

5. Make sure your work surfaces are at a comfortable height.

6. Never lean on objects. Stand straight on your own two feet.

7. If you are tall, don't stoop. Be proud of your height.

8. Your feet play an important part in good posture. Take good care of them! (See section on feet.)

Remember that, with concentration and perseverance, good posture can be attained. Good posture is always a mark of glowing good health, glamour, and beauty.

the importance of breathing correctly

Feeling tired, nervous, uptight? Take a deep breath. It's one of the most relaxing and energizing things you can do. Try taking a deep breath right now. Feel how new energy spreads throughout your body. Now exhale. Feel the tiredness and the poisonous substances leaving your body. Breathing is such an easy, natural, and healthful thing to do. It's distressing that most people do not know how to do it correctly!

Correct deep breathing is, sad to say, a lost art, and breathing is the basis of all normal activities for all living things; for human beings it is the most crucial. It affects our state of health, our mental condition, our very lifespan. We can live days without solid food, but we can live only a few minutes without air.

Primitive man did not have to learn the art of correct breathing. His lifestyle assured it. Fresh air, a natural environment, continual movement, a wide variety of natural physical activities, and the struggle for survival with the elements made early man a good breather. Civilized man, however, lives a life far removed from all these components of natural life and physical activity. And one of the prices modern man pays for civilization is anxiety, probably the single greatest reason man has "forgotten" how to breathe correctly.

Every so often nature tries to help us return to a refreshed, relaxed, natural state. Without thinking about it, we stretch and breathe when we have been in one position too long, yawn when we are tired, or sigh when we feel that life has become too much of a burden for us. These are nature's ways of compelling us to take a good deep breath when we really need one.

The purpose of deep, rhythmic breathing is to help us take greater amounts of oxygen into our lungs and then expel all the stale, used-up air in the form of carbon dioxide. These two actions, intake and expulsion, recharge the bloodstream and improve circulation. Good circulation adds new energy and vitality.

Thinking becomes clearer and movement becomes easier and more graceful.

We bring oxygen into the body in many ways. The nose, the nasal passages, the pharynx, larynx, and bronchial tubes are the primary ways. The nostrils filter dust particles from the incoming air. The mucous membrane of the nose, with its bacteria, secretes mucus which helps purify incoming air and rid it of germs.

Filtered and tempered air is carried to the lungs by the bronchial tubes, which divide into a great many cells, each with corresponding capillary blood vessels. These radiate through the body, absorbing fresh oxygen and eliminating carbonic acid. The freshly oxygenated blood travels from the lungs to the heart, and from there is sent to all parts of the body. When the blood returns to the lungs, the bloodstream is charged with carbonic acid which is ready to be eliminated. This continuous circulatory system is so complex and ingenious as to be one of the most incredible functions of the human body.

During shallow respiration the lung cells do not work hard enough to ensure a complete change of oxygen and carbonic acid. Wastes are not completely expelled and these can accumulate in the system and create unpleasant toxic effects. This becomes especially troublesome as we grow older because, with advancing age, the lungs and thorax are apt to lose their elasticity, and their full and proper functioning becomes impaired. For this reason alone, correct breathing is of vital importance.

Yet there are other reasons too. Breathing is most important to health and beauty and it is an important technique of Body Rhythms. Correctly done, proper breathing brings the muscles of the neck, shoulders, and chest into play, and increases circulation as well. When we are active, our muscles need more air to perform their stepped-up functioning.

When resting, we breathe about fifteen times a minute, and each breath exchanges a pint of air. This may seem an adequate amount, but when we take only a slightly longer and deeper breath, see what happens: we exchange three pints of air. With a still longer and deeper breath, six pints of air enter the lungs. Expanded to their fullest, adult lungs have a possible content of about three and one-half quarts of air! In shallow breathing we exchange only a tiny fraction of the possible air content of our lungs. When we walk, the air content of our lungs increases two

and one-half times over the amount they contain while we are resting. Mountain climbing raises this figure to ten times. And when we swim, our lungs are expanded twenty times more than when we are at rest.

Normally, air is a mixture of oxygen and nitrogen plus a small amount of other chemicals. Very often, however, it is also filled with dust, soot, noxious gases, and countless other destructive particles. When we breathe through the mouth—an all-too-frequent bad habit—no filtering process takes place, as it does when air is inhaled through the nose. Because the nasal filtering process is so important, it is vital to keep the nasal passages as clear as possible at all times so that the cilia, or small hairs, can help to remove foreign objects, and the mucus can combat bacteria.

Deep breathing is a form of exercise you can start doing right away. When you do it, try to wear nothing that binds or restricts the free movement of your chest. Whenever possible, practice outdoors. If you must be indoors, breathe near an open window.

The best way to practice deep breathing is in conjunction with Body Rhythms. But it is also possible to practice breathing wherever you are: as you ride up or down in an elevator, stand in line at the supermarket, wait for a bus or train. If you make a habit of deep breathing at these times, you'll be rewarded with increased vitality and stamina.

the three methods of breathing

There are three methods of breathing. Properly, they should all be used together. The first, "high breath," is, unfortunately, the kind of shallow breathing done by most people: only the upper portion of the lungs is brought into play. This method, alone, is entirely insufficient. Many women are restricted in their breathing by wearing tight girdles, as well as by the amount of time they spend sitting in soft chairs, hunched over their work. This shallow and superficial pattern of breathing is occasionally interrupted by a deeper breath, such as a yawn—the desperate reflex of air-thirsty lungs!

The "medium," or "costal," breath is an improvement on the first type of breathing. During costal breathing the lungs are filled to the middle, the ribs are activated and expanded, rising while the diaphragm lowers. Most men breathe this way, and more women should consciously try to learn to do so, as a step toward correct, full breathing. Costal breathing should be practiced while standing—action should come from the ribs, which rise when you inhale. Practiced slowly and rhythmically, this type of breathing can keep the chest muscles elastic. Costal breathing is also an excellent aid in developing the bosom and helps prevent rigidity in the entire chest area as one grows older. Moreover, this deeper breathing is considered an excellent means of preventing colds and other chest illnesses.

Best of all is abdominal or diaphragm breathing, which fills both the lower and middle lungs with air. This third method is recommended by many health specialists as an excellent practice. You can do abdominal breathing lying flat on your back. Inhale, trying to extend the abdomen to the utmost while keeping your chest in a fixed position. Now contract and flatten the abdomen as far as possible and breathe out slowly. This type of breathing activates internal organs, increases circulation, and helps in the digestion and assimilation of food.

Proper breathing should combine all three Though hard to master, a complete and proper breath should combine all three methods described above. This takes practice and nearly perfect muscle control. The entire breathing apparatus, every cell of the lungs, all the muscles involved, are brought into action. Begin by standing straight with legs slightly apart. Exhale completely. Then, inhaling through the nose, begin with the abdominal breath. Activate the diaphragm, pushing the abdomen outward. This automatically fills the lower part of the lungs with air. Then expand the lower ribs and middle thorax region, gradually taking in air from the lower part of the lungs. Correct breathing process starts from the base and moves upward—not, as is commonly thought, from the neck down. Finally, try to attain a complete expansion of the thorax. Take in as much air as you can into your fully expanded lungs, drawing in the abdomen as support for the lungs. Exhale slowly in the same succession. Draw in the abdomen, contract the ribs, relax your collarbone and shoulders.

Correct breathing should never be tiring. On the contrary, it is a refresher and should energize the entire body. When strengthened, the diaphragm assumes its proper function and plays an important part in breathing. Correct breathing also exerts slight pressure on the liver, stomach, and digestive tract and acts as a mild massage.

Both costal and abdominal breathing systems are necessary for perfect physical health. They are interrelated, each affecting the other. If you are able to make them work together, the increased intake of oxygen can bring a speedier breakdown of fat cells—a big help to the woman with an overweight problem. They can also expand and develop the chest, building underlying tissues which support the breast; thus they are of equal benefit to the underweight and flat-chested.

In my teaching experience I have found that most people are apt to hold their breaths or breathe spasmodically when exercising. Consequently, all benefits to be derived from the exercise are lost. Nervous tension, unnecessary exertion, and loss of energy are the results.

The knowledge and practice of natural, deep, rhythmic breathing are a must. It is a great achievement to become aware of an important function that you have so long taken for granted. Take another deep breath. Exhale. It might help you to count: six counts to inhale, six to retain, six to exhale. You might gradually increase the count to eight, nine, or ten. The things to bear in mind are: to establish a tempo, perhaps in time with your pulse beat; to relax as you breathe; to think of it as a natural, easy function.

If you are willing to concentrate on correcting your breathing faults for even a few days, you will find that correct breathing will become a part of your daily living schedule.

relaxation
— relieving stress,
tension, anxiety

Stress . . . tension . . . anxiety. We know these words only too well. They are practically synonymous with modern living. The twentieth century is a time of maximum pressure and minimum relaxation. When was the last time you just sat quietly and did nothing, for example? Or communed with nature? Chances are it was so long ago that you can't even remember!

Signs of this modern malaise are all around us. Just have a look at the people you pass as you hurry down the street. City expressions are hard; faces are pinched tightly with worry and anxiety. Bodies are bent forward with urgency and drive. Feet move at a rapid tempo. Voices are harsh, tempers are short, and patience is a forgotten word!

People in small cities and towns are more fortunate. They know what it's like to relax, to move about one's business naturally, to take the time to think and contemplate. City people are not so lucky. Since our lives seem to preclude free moments for ourselves, we must make a conscious effort to make the time. We must escape from the constant pressure, noise, and harassment. In short, we simply must learn how to relax.

As women, we are perhaps the most obvious victims of this stress–tension–anxiety syndrome—in terms of femininity lost and hardened faces gained. But it is quite possible for us to be islands of peace and tranquillity, putting an end to this mass of nervous tension and minimizing its wasting effects. By doing so, we can do a great service to ourselves and others.

Tension takes a high toll from our nervous systems and our sense of well-being. Its symptoms attack health, beauty, and peace of mind. Sleeplessness, headaches, digestive disturbances, overwhelming fatigue, irritability and extreme nervousness are all symptoms of tension. A destroyer of poise and charm—of everything even the most "liberated" woman should be—tension can make you an impossible person for others to live with, and an impossible companion even for yourself.

the body's major tension areas

Tension derives not from overused, but from underutilized muscles, which become inflexible through inactivity. The areas where your body tenses and stiffens most are the *back of the neck* and the *upper part of the spine*, the *lumbar or lower spinal region,* and the *backs of the knees.* This is because these areas are never used in daily activities unless you deliberately make them active.

The back of the neck and upper part of the spine The back of the neck is where tension accumulates more than in any other place. Most people droop their heads forward when they stand or sit, which rounds the upper vertebrae. Unless this poor posture habit is counteracted, the muscles become hard and taut, impede blood circulation, and cause that familiar pain at the back of the neck that so many people complain about constantly. Special corrective exercises for the neck area will counteract this difficulty (see Body Rhythms 7–10). Learning how to eliminate this tension may take a little time and patience, but the effort is definitely worthwhile.

The lower back The lower back is particularly vulnerable. Few people use the lower back, tending to move the torso from the waist or upper shoulders rather than from the hip joints. Unless you do very special exercises, the lower back is rarely in action; tension develops in the spinal column, and primarily in the lumbar region. When the back is stiff and rigid, the abdomen spreads and develops bulges. Women try to hide these bulges with girdles that only add to their troubles by impeding circulation and active participation of the body's major muscles, especially those of the abdomen, waist, lower back, thighs, and hips. When these become weak and rigid they cause lower back pains. It is of utmost importance to strengthen these muscles to

These thorough stretching and relaxing movements are wonderful for tense, taut, and tired bodies. After a few stretches back and forth the body feels relaxed, refreshed, and alive again.

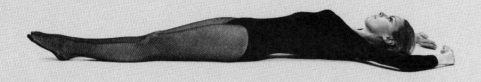

Lie on the floor with arms relaxed above head, knees straight, toes pointed.

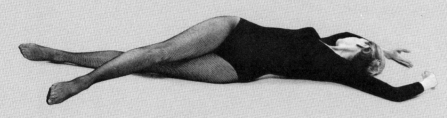

Breathe in, lift right thigh and leg and stretch toward left. Stretch upper part of body — head, arm and shoulder — from the waistline in the opposite direction.

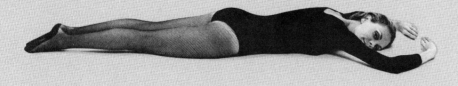

Breathe out and roll body over facing down.

Breathe in, lift head, left arm, and shoulder stretching toward right, from the waistline. Stretch left thigh and leg in the opposite direction.

Breathe out and roll body over facing up. Relax.

Alternate movement from right to left and left to right.

Repeat five times.

prevent them from slackening. There is no way of putting them into condition except through corrective exercises geared specifically for the lower back (see Body Rhythms 1–6, 16–18).

The backs of the knees The backs of the knees are another problem area where tension accumulates and shrinks muscles. In the sitting position, the outside muscles of the thigh and leg are stretched, but the inside and back muscles are not. Also, continual wearing of high heels shrinks the back of the calf and the knee. To counteract this tension, it is also necessary to do special exercises to stretch the muscles in the back of the leg, the calf, and the knee (see Body Rhythms 1–6, 19–21).

If you don't exercise properly to learn how to relax tension, it keeps accumulating all the time. This is why so many people reach the point where they can't take it any longer and must go on vacation. They may not realize why they're so tired. Tension makes you tired; and if you don't know how to rid your body of stress and tension, you'll be constantly tired.

One big mistake people make is to try to dispel tension by getting too much sleep and rest. This is the worst thing in the world; the more you try to rest, the worse you feel. Inactivity only adds to tension and fatigue. The remedy is to limber up your body by exercising correctly.

body rhythms – active exercise to relieve tension

The key, of course, to relief of tension is relaxation, and it is something you must train yourself to do. Most people don't realize how tense they are until they have learned to relax and to use their bodies correctly. Real relaxation can only come about when your body is completely limber in every joint, muscle, ligament, and nerve. This can best be achieved through Body Rhythms—the right type of anatomically correct exercises which stretch you thoroughly and make you feel refreshed and relaxed at the end of each session. To rid the body of tension, you have to stretch slowly, breathe deeply, and completely relax when you finish each movement.

Proper deep breathing is a very important adjunct to Body Rhythms. By inhaling deeply and exhaling completely, you not only fill your lungs with fresh air and expel all the stale air, but you relax your body automatically at the same time. Breathe in deeply through your nose and breathe out completely through your mouth. Remember that when you stretch in Body Rhythms you inhale, and as you relax, you exhale. This will eventually come so naturally you will hardly realize you are doing it.

Begin by relaxing with a hot bath Instead of exercising immediately when you get home after a busy day, it is better to lie in a hot bath for about ten minutes first. Heat relaxes the body and helps rid it of tension. Then you're in better condition for stretching and deep breathing. After the hot bath and exercise, take a rest.

massage — passive exercise to relieve tension

Massage is a passive substitute for exercise and gives wonderfully beneficial side effects. Its gentle manipulation is soothing, restful, and health-giving. Massage does not reduce weight, however, to any appreciable degree, as is commonly believed.

Many people erroneously think that the manipulation of muscle tissues will break up unwanted fat deposits, which will then be carried away by the bloodstream. This is nonsense! It has been proven that a pressure of fifty to seventy-five pounds per square inch would have to be exerted in order to actually break up fat cells. If such pressure were to be applied by a masseuse or a machine, the injury to tissues would be irreparable. Whenever massage is undertaken, care must always be exercised to prevent deep bruising of the muscle tissue. If properly administered, massage can be an excellent aid in stimulating circulation, eliminating tension, and relaxing the body as a whole.

Historical records from even the earliest of civilizations have shown how massage was used to relieve pain. One of the most commonly employed therapeutic measures is the almost instinctive application of a kneading and stroking motion to an area as soon as acute pain is experienced. Ancient in origin, massage was known to the pharaohs of Egypt and was practiced by the Romans. As it found favor in various countries, each contributed its own local innovations, producing such variations as the Swedish, Danish, and Russian massage systems. All are built upon the same basic movements of stroking, compression, and percussion. The small differences from country to country are not of particular therapeutic significance. It can be said, however, that massage, if administered in one way, has a sedative effect on the nervous system, and, if applied in another way, has a stimulating effect. In either case, it works by stepping up the circulation of the bloodstream through the reflex stimulation of the muscles and the mechanical compression of the blood vessels.

To administer massage effectively, one must have some knowledge of anatomy and physiology, as well as of techniques of massage. It is my firm belief that unless you can get massage administered by an experienced operator, you are better off without any. The clumsy pounding and hacking of the body by an inept person can be nerve-racking, harmful, and unhealthy. Any competent masseuse knows when massage is not recommended. Never should it be performed over inflamed, swollen, or arthritic joints, over sprains, or over severe bruises where there might be internal bleeding. Increased circulation to these areas would only add more fluid to the injury. Massage tends, also, to spread acute infections; therefore, such conditions as boils, carbuncles, or infected wounds should never be touched. In some cases there are even toxic reactions to increased circulation. Neither should massage be prescribed for anyone suffering from a debilitating disease or for an older person with high blood pressure. And wherever there is even the slightest suspicion of a skin disorder or a swelling, a person should not be massaged unless it is on the advice of a physician.

An experienced operator will use her palms, not her fingers, in administering massage. Working upward, her movements begin with a gentle, firm stroking, followed by deep kneading pressure on the upward sweep only, becoming gentle as the hands move downward. Any pressure in the movement should be aimed at assisting the flow of blood in the veins; therefore, it should be applied in a direction toward the heart.

Tense, large muscle groups are helped in their relaxation by the compression movements of massage. After circulation has been stimulated by deep stroking, the next step is the kneading of the fleshy portions of the body. The masseuse lifts and compresses the tissue in a movement similar to that of kneading dough. The amount of pressure she uses should be in proportion to the tone or tenseness of the muscle. Flabby muscles can be further weakened and even injured if too much pressure is used. If the muscles, in general, are well-developed and healthy, percussive movements may be administered to increase circulation.

Caution: The one area that should not be massaged is the breasts. Even a gentle massage can cause irritation and congestion in these glands.

Is a self-administered massage possible?   Some physical experts recommend a "do-it-yourself" massage. It is my strong conviction that it is impossible and an absolutely worthless effort. Since massage is primarily for the purpose of complete relaxation, anything you do yourself will add tension and fatigue rather than eliminate them. I therefore do not advise self-administered massage—it isn't restful and it isn't relaxing.

To those of you who have never contemplated massage before, it may seem an extravagant form of self-indulgence, without special value. It isn't. Your first experience will easily convince you that the restful and luxurious feeling following a massage is easily worth the time and expense. Especially when you are overtired or tense, its benefits are significant. You will sit up feeling refreshed, relaxed, and renewed. You'll wonder why you didn't try it sooner.

what can you expect in 10 days?

In the previous sections I discussed the importance of altering lifelong bad habits and making lifelong commitments for improved health, energy, and beauty. Now it is time to get down to the specifics of the Body Rhythms program. You may well wonder whether adhering to this plan for only ten days can actually make a significant difference. The answer is: yes, absolutely. The human body—and the mind—are marvelously adaptable—adapting is in fact one of the things we do best.

The Body Rhythms program is divided into three parts. The first consists of those exercises you will undertake in the 10-Day Health and Beauty Program. The Intermediate and Advanced movements are those you will work up to, slowly, one by one, in the days that follow. The next section discusses diet and nutrition, subjects of related importance if the body is to develop and maintain health and vigor, and especially if weight is a problem.

In examining these sections you will learn how to design for yourself the exact health and figure correction program your body needs. You will learn how, and why, to follow an energizing diet, as well as how to eliminate or prevent back pain and how to improve posture. You will learn how to keep the muscles of your face and neck firm and youthful-looking for many years to come.

Who stands to benefit?   For the woman who has no weight problem, the 10-Day Health and Beauty Program could be sufficient to reshape the body to graceful, ideal proportions, provided it is followed by a modest but regular schedule of exercise, and is supplemented by a sensible, nutritious diet. The body will thrive and continue to improve.

For the woman who has a weight problem, there is no doubt that the intensive 10-Day program will give amazing results in loss of weight and inches. However, do not expect miracles if your body is extremely overweight. This will take time; certainly

This table illustrates how the Manya Kahn Body Rhythms system takes inches off where they are unwanted and leaves them where they are needed. Each client worked on her particular problem at her own pace —from ten days to one year. Body Rhythms, correct nutrition, and learning how to relax enabled them to achieve their goals.

The most exciting thing about the Manya Kahn program is that during the process of losing weight the skin gradually adjusts itself to the new measurements while the muscles tone up and firm. This amazing transformation is long lasting and often permanent.

MEASUREMENTS (in inches)

		WEIGHT	arm	neck	bust	diaph.	waist	hips	both thighs	thigh	knee	calf	ankle
M.K. 5'5" model													
10 days/10sessions/everyday	before	109	9	12	31	25½	25½	34	37½	22½	14	12¾	8
	after	99	8½	11½	31	24½	23	31½	35	20	13½	12½	7¾
E.R. 5'7" fashion director													
1 month/10 sessions/3 times week	before	136	10¾	12	33	29	26	35	40	25¾	17	15½	9¾
	after	134	10¾	12	33	29	26	35	37	22½	15½	15	9¼
J.H. 5'4½" bank executive													
1 month/10 sessions/3 times week	before	131	11½	12½	33	28	27¼	35	40	24½	16	14	8¾
	after	121	10½	12	32½	27	25¾	33½	38	23	15	13	8¼
S.K. 5'8" writer													
5 weeks/15 sessions/3 times week	before	125	9	13¼	32½	25½	24¾	35	34¾	20½	13¾	11¼	8½
	after	133	10	14	34	26½	24	36	37	21½	14	12½	8½
J.G. 5'4" medical researcher													
6 weeks/20 sessions/3–4 times week	before	127	10¼	12¾	32	28½	25½	34	39	24	15	14	9
	after	113	10	12	33	27	24¼	33	35¾	21½	14¼	13½	8½

MEASUREMENTS (in inches)

		WEIGHT	arm	neck	bust	diaph.	waist	hips	both thighs	thigh	knee	calf	ankle
J.C. 5'7"													
psychologist	before	159¾	12¾	14	37	28	28	41	45	26½	17	17	9
2 months/20 sessions/3 times week	after	138	11¼	11¾	34	27	26½	35½	38½	23½	17	16¼	8¼
A.Z. 5'7"													
teacher	before	150	11¾	12¾	36½	30½	29¾	38	42	24¾	17	14½	9¼
2 months/20 sessions/3 times week	after	131	10½	12½	34¼	27½	26¾	34½	38	22	15	14	8½
W.J. 5'9"													
socialite	after 3 mos. 165 before	165	13	14	38	32	32	40	42	26	17	15	10
socialite	after 3 mos.	148	12	13¾	36½	30	29½	38	38½	24½	15¾	13¾	9¼
6 months/100 sessions/4–5 times week	after 6 mos.	131¾	11	13¼	34	28	27	35½	36	22½	15	12¾	9
M.V.B. 5'6"													
socialite	before	144	12	12¾	36½	32	32¼	41	41	25	15¾	13½	8½
6 months/50 sessions/3,4,5 times week	after	123	11	12½	33	28	27	35½	36	21½	14¼	13	7¾
P.R. 5'5"													
teacher	before	155	11½	13	35	30	30	41	45	28	18	15	9
1 year/50 sessions/2 times week	after	123	9½	11½	33	25½	25½	35½	38½	23	16	14½	8¾

more than ten days, but the first ten days will serve as the inspiration to continue on this program until your goal is reached. (The table on pages 32–33 shows conclusive proof of what determination and effort can achieve.)

The woman who is underweight and underdeveloped can also benefit from the intensive 10-Day program. By following the specific diets outlined in the diet section, you will begin to build muscle tissue, increase your stamina and vitality, and you will get rid of tension and fatigue—so often the cause of the inability to assimilate food. By following the Body Rhythms program consistently and carefully, the increase in poundage will settle on the parts of the body most needed for feminine curves.

how to perform body rhythms for best results

To perform Body Rhythms all you need is a leotard and a pair of tights—freshly laundered each time you wear them!—a thick floor mat or firm mattress.

At my salon I have developed the slantboard, a padded, six-foot board that allows you to elevate your feet at a 20-degree angle. Circulation of the blood is thus encouraged in the upper part of the body. By reversing the upright position of the body, the blood flows into the neck and muscle tissues of the face, thereby stimulating the skin and enhancing the complexion.

If you are unable to obtain a slantboard, you can build one or have one built like the one illustrated here. Under no circumstances should you work on a board that collapses in the center or one without sufficient padding—at least 3 inches thick.

If you have a weak back and weak abdominal muscles, you should definitely plan to use the slantboard, for lifting the legs from the flat surface of the floor is difficult and uncomfortable.

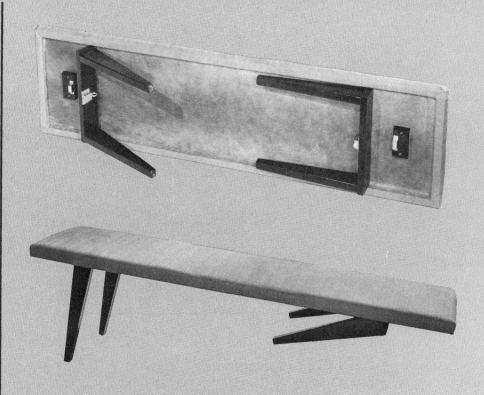

The slantboard will enable you to obtain results quickly on the 10-Day Program. As shown, the slantboard has two sets of folding legs 14 inches high and is constructed with a solid board 66–72 inches long by 20 inches wide. It is padded with a 3-inch-thick foam mattress and covered with a rough-finish fabric.

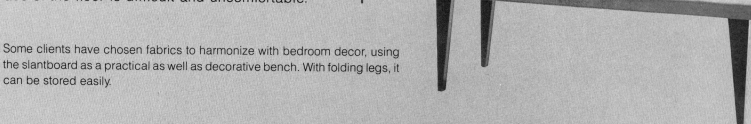

Some clients have chosen fabrics to harmonize with bedroom decor, using the slantboard as a practical as well as decorative bench. With folding legs, it can be stored easily.

34

The slantboard is not a necessity, but be sure to avoid a too-soft or too-hard surface. If you use a mat, it should be firm, 3 inches thick. Working directly on a hard floor can do actual damage to the spinal column.

when to perform body rhythms

You can exercise anytime at your convenience, except directly after meals: you should wait at least an hour and a half to allow time for digestion. If you exercise in the morning, you will find Body Rhythms bracing and stimulating. If you exercise at night, Body Rhythms will help you relax and sleep better.

If you practice indoors, the windows should be open to provide good ventilation. Remember that breathing must be carefully coordinated. Inhale deeply through your nose as you begin each movement and exhale slowly as you complete the movement. Deep inhaling and exhaling will fill the lungs with fresh air and will expel stale air.

Work daily—an hour at a time The number of Body Rhythms performed daily depends upon your own stamina and vitality. As a general rule, it is best to work up to the suggested regimen gradually. *Remember:* quality is more important than quantity. Concentrate on proper execution. Body Rhythms should be practiced with slow—smooth—flowing motions, s-t-r-e-t-c-h-i-n-g each part of your body as far as you can without strain. Never exercise at the expense of your energy. As soon as you begin to feel tired, *stop.*

I must stress, however, that during the 10-Day program, Body Rhythms must be performed *daily* and *consistently.* You must not skip a single day. No, you cannot make up for missing a day by working twice as hard the next day, no more than you can overeat one day and starve the next. If you intend to exercise only occasionally when a burst of enthusiasm comes over you, beware of disappointing results.

Follow body rhythms with a bath or shower A bath or a shower after a Body Rhythms session is necessary because the body must be cleansed of the impurities thrown off through the pores during exercising. A bath refreshes the skin, and at the same time you can perform other beauty rituals important to a well-groomed woman.

If you practice in the morning, a shower is recommended; if you practice in the evening before going to bed, Body Rhythms should be followed by a warm, soothing bath.

Some women have found that exercising works wonders after a busy day. If this works best for you, a hot bath should be taken beforehand. Heat relaxes the body and helps rid it of tension. Then you're in better condition for stretching and deep breathing. After the bath and exercise, take a rest.

I hope you are convinced by now that everyone needs to take positive steps to maintain or to improve the body. The accompanying chart will show you how to measure yourself, providing you with a 10-Day, 6-Month, 10-Year Calendar of weight and measurements achieved through the Manya Kahn Body Rhythms program.

After the concentrated 10-Day program you will not only have toned up your body significantly by strengthening the entire muscle structure, you will have learned correct breathing and improved posture, and you will be able to practice, without thinking, every day. A steady maintenance program is essential. If a daily schedule is impossible, then you should practice at least three times a week for an hour—you can split the program into two half hours: thirty minutes in the morning and thirty minutes in the evening.

Your body will reward you with increased energy, a palpable sense of well-being, and you will become noticeably and increasingly more attractive.

The Manya Kahn system works, and after only ten days you will know it works, beyond question.

manya kahn weight and measurement chart

At the beginning of the 10-Day program, measure yourself in the exact spots illustrated and record your measurements. Weigh yourself daily on the same scale—same time each day—and record your weight. Make every effort to be exact, for only an accurate weight and measurement record can help you make necessary diet or exercise adjustments. After ten days, measure yourself again, and compare the wonderful results!

Whatever your problem—overweight, underweight, or out of shape—you will have gained the incentive for continued work on your problem. The chart provides for a reevaluation in six months and again after a year, plus space for analysis over a ten-year period.

Before starting on your reshaping program, please check with your physician. This is particularly important in order to rule out any suspicion that your problem may be due to some organic or glandular disturbance.

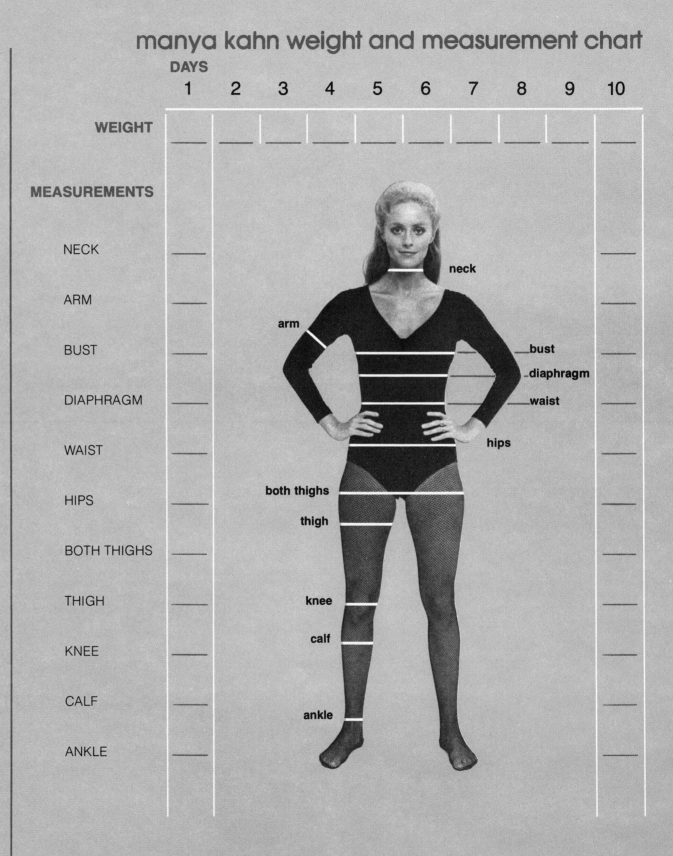

DAYS

	1	2	3	4	5	6	7	8	9	10
WEIGHT										
MEASUREMENTS										
NECK										
ARM										
BUST										
DIAPHRAGM										
WAIST										
HIPS										
BOTH THIGHS										
THIGH										
KNEE										
CALF										
ANKLE										

after six months	after one year	YEARS 2	3	4	5	6	7	8	9	10	
_____	_____	_____	_____	_____	_____	_____	_____	_____	_____	_____	**WEIGHT**
											MEASUREMENTS
_____	_____	_____	_____	_____	_____	_____	_____	_____	_____	_____	NECK
_____	_____	_____	_____	_____	_____	_____	_____	_____	_____	_____	ARM
_____	_____	_____	_____	_____	_____	_____	_____	_____	_____	_____	BUST
_____	_____	_____	_____	_____	_____	_____	_____	_____	_____	_____	DIAPHRAGM
_____	_____	_____	_____	_____	_____	_____	_____	_____	_____	_____	WAIST
_____	_____	_____	_____	_____	_____	_____	_____	_____	_____	_____	HIPS
_____	_____	_____	_____	_____	_____	_____	_____	_____	_____	_____	BOTH THIGHS
_____	_____	_____	_____	_____	_____	_____	_____	_____	_____	_____	THIGH
_____	_____	_____	_____	_____	_____	_____	_____	_____	_____	_____	KNEE
_____	_____	_____	_____	_____	_____	_____	_____	_____	_____	_____	CALF
_____	_____	_____	_____	_____	_____	_____	_____	_____	_____	_____	ANKLE

manya kahn body rhythms

basic body rhythms

body rhythms to stretch spine, strengthen lumbar region and firm abdomen (1-6)

Body Rhythms are a progressive series of triple-action movements that must be performed in sequence.

Work on a slantboard, if possible; if not, work on a mat at least two or three inches thick.

Practice with slow rhythms coordinated with deep breathing.

Always remember:

1 Keep lower back flat against slant-board.
2 Keep abdomen pulled in.
3 Keep back of knees flat against slantboard.
4 Keep feet flexed to stretch muscles in back of legs.
5 Keep buttocks firm as legs are lowered to Starting Position.

When directions are given to "bounce three times," it means to move about four inches back and forth.

STARTING POSITION
Lie flat on slantboard with lower part of back touching board, knees straight, arms at sides, hands grasping board, toes pointed.

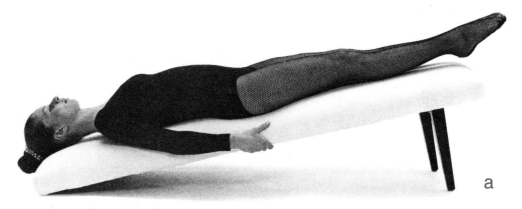

a

From Starting Position, flex both feet, bringing toes toward you, pushing heels out to straighten knees.

Breathe in while you stretch both arms out sideways, then back, stretching elbows and fingers at the same time. Hold for one second.

Breathe out while returning slowly to Starting Position. Relax.

Repeat five times.

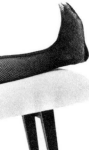

b

40

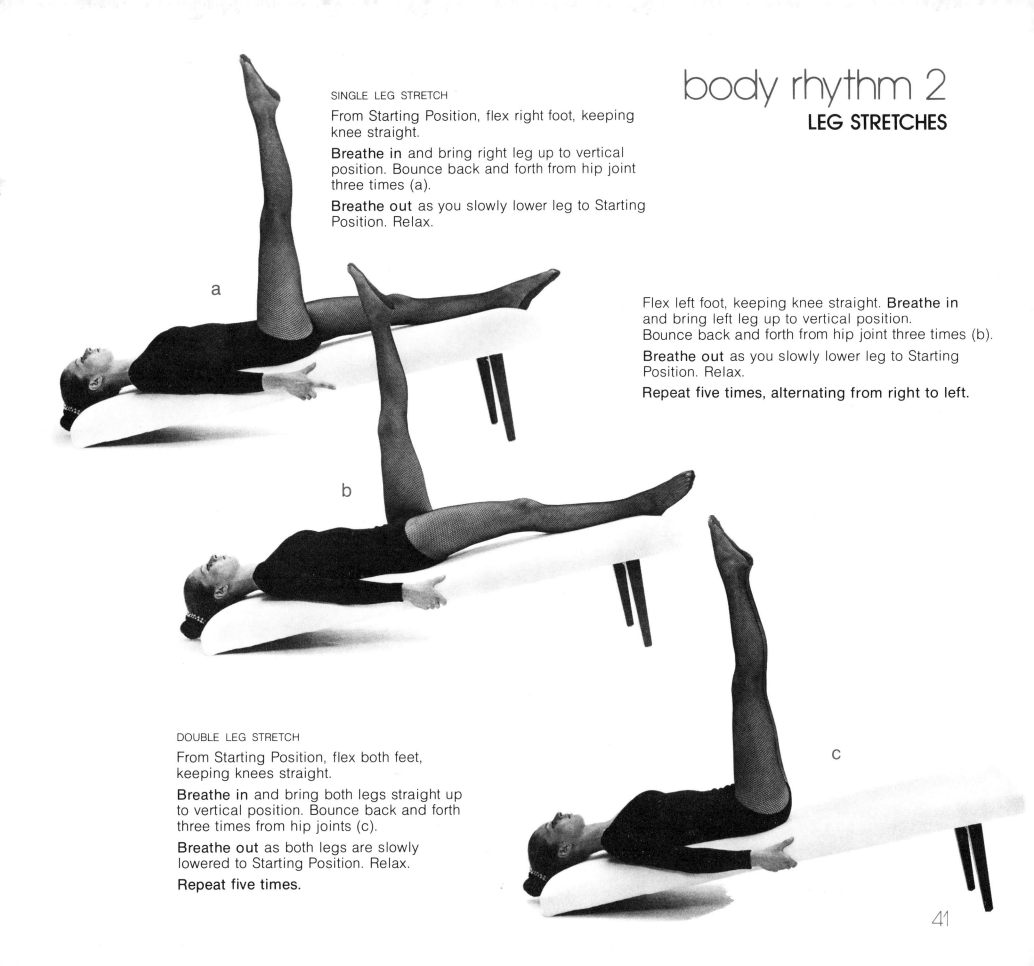

SINGLE LEG STRETCH

From Starting Position, flex right foot, keeping knee straight.

Breathe in and bring right leg up to vertical position. Bounce back and forth from hip joint three times (a).

Breathe out as you slowly lower leg to Starting Position. Relax.

Flex left foot, keeping knee straight. **Breathe in** and bring left leg up to vertical position. Bounce back and forth from hip joint three times (b).

Breathe out as you slowly lower leg to Starting Position. Relax.

Repeat five times, alternating from right to left.

DOUBLE LEG STRETCH

From Starting Position, flex both feet, keeping knees straight.

Breathe in and bring both legs straight up to vertical position. Bounce back and forth three times from hip joints (c).

Breathe out as both legs are slowly lowered to Starting Position. Relax.

Repeat five times.

41

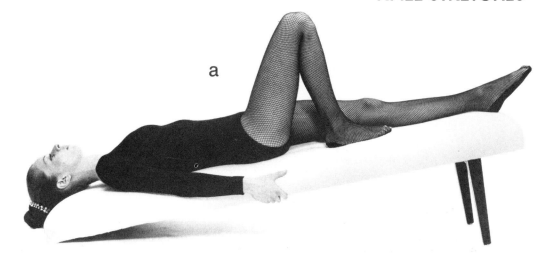

a

From Starting Position, **breathe in,** bend right knee, placing foot flat on slantboard (a).

Breathe out, bring knee into chest. Bounce knee back and forth toward chest three times from hip joint (b).

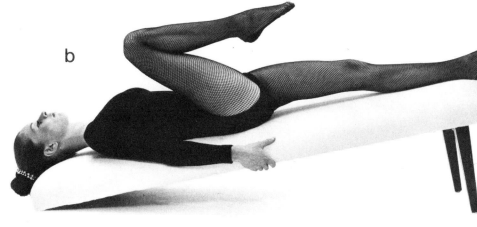

b

Breathe in as you stretch leg straight up, toes pointed (c).

Flex foot and bring leg slowly down as you **breathe out.**

Repeat with left leg.

Do each movement five times, alternating from right to left.

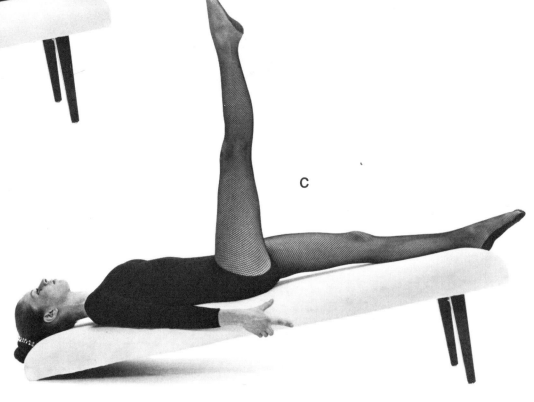

c

42

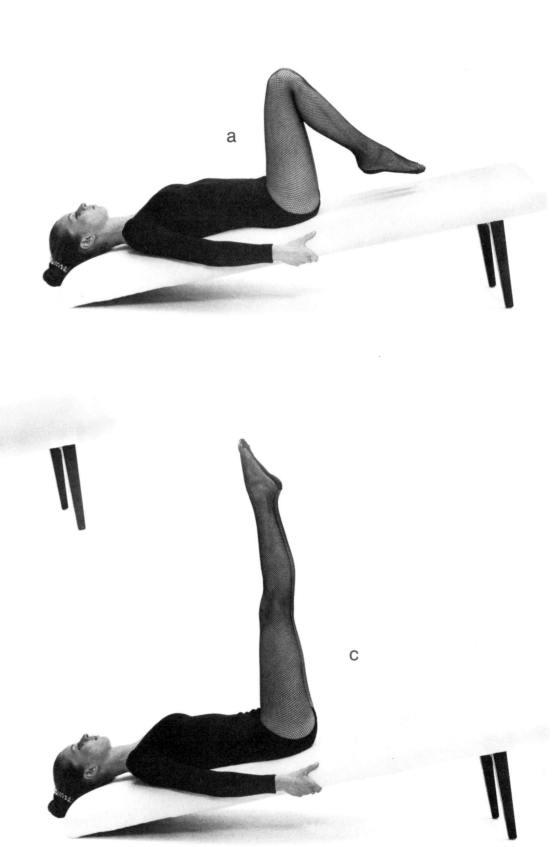

DOUBLE KNEE STRETCH

From Starting Position, **breathe in,** bend both knees (a), placing feet flat on slantboard.

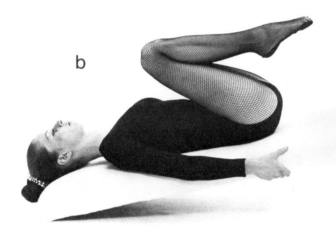

Breathe out, bring both knees into chest. Bounce knees back and forth toward chest three times from hip joints (b).

Breathe in, stretch both legs straight up with toes pointed, knees straight (c). Flex both feet, bring both legs slowly down as you **breathe out.** Relax.

Repeat five times.

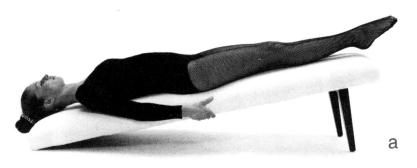

a

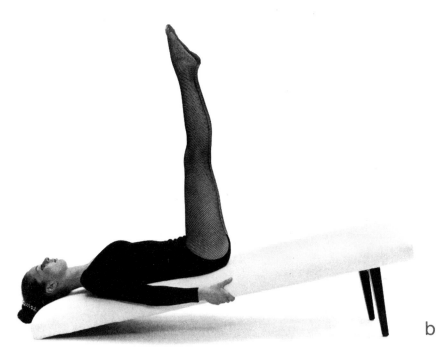

b

From Starting Position (a) flex both feet. **Breathe in** as you lift both legs straight up to vertical position, keeping knees as straight as possible (b).

Breathe out as you stretch legs wide apart. Bounce legs three times from hip joints.

Breathe in as you bring both legs back to center (d), still in a vertical position.

Breathe out as you slowly lower both legs down to Starting Position. Relax.

As you practice the Inner Thigh Stretch, gradually widen the stretch as you limber the inner thigh muscles (e).

Repeat five times.

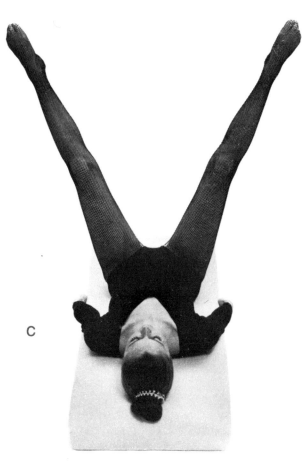

c

44

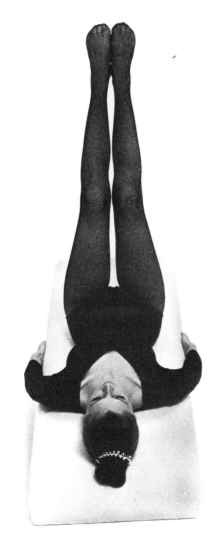

d

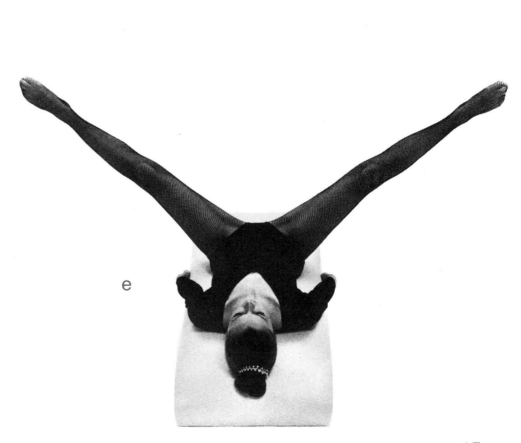

e

45

From Starting Position (a), flex both feet. **Breathe in** as you lift both legs straight up to vertical position, keeping knees as straight as possible (b).

Breathe out as you stretch both legs wide apart (c), then slowly circle out and down (d) to Starting Position (e). Relax.

Reverse. **Breathe in,** stretch legs out and up (f, g), circling back to vertical position (h). **Breathe out.** Lower slowly to Starting Position. Relax.

Repeat circles in both directions five times.

body rhythm 5
SINGLE LEG CIRCLES

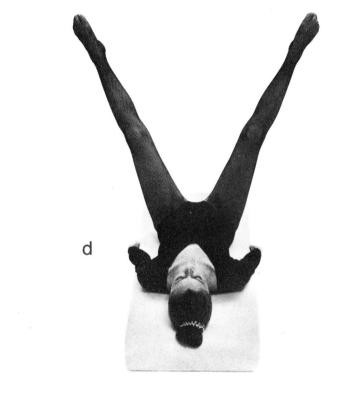

d

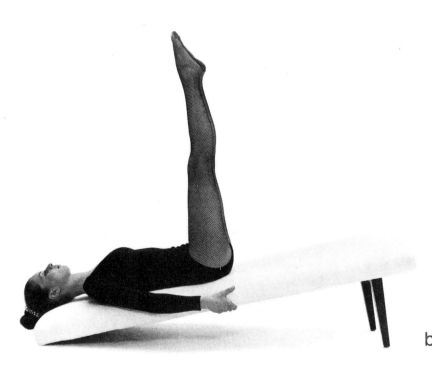

a

b

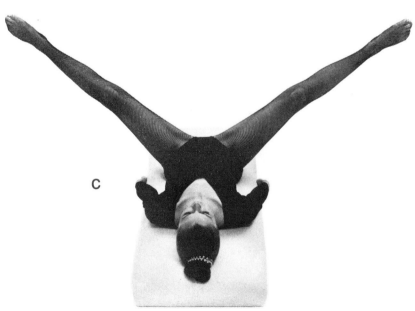

c

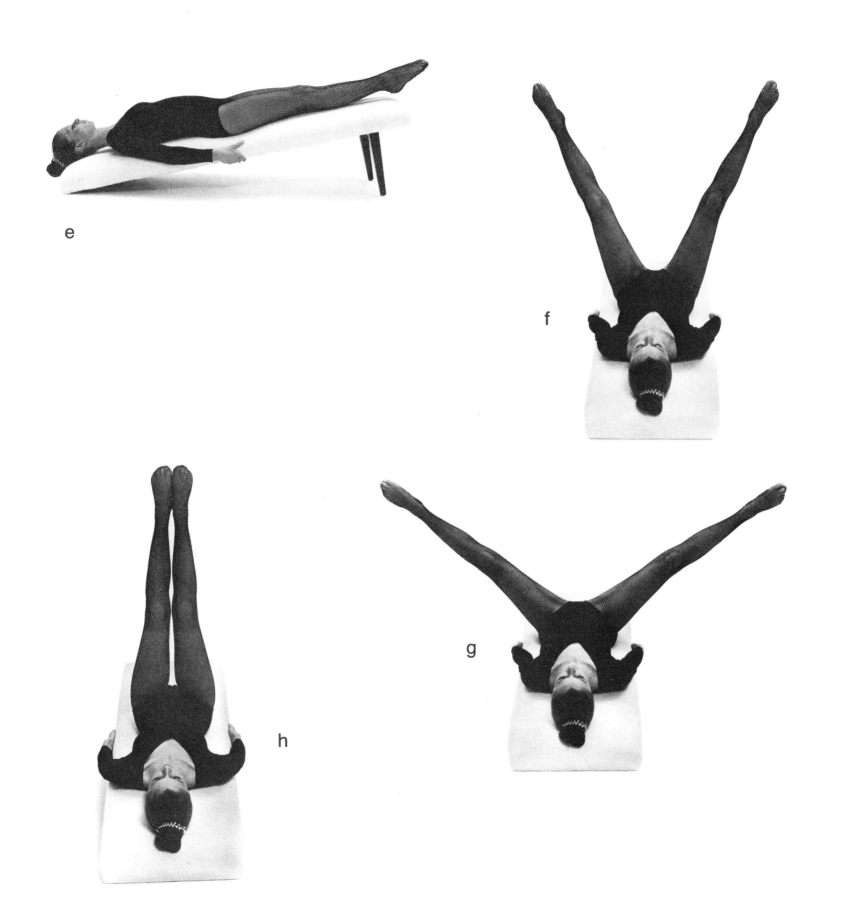

e

f

g

h

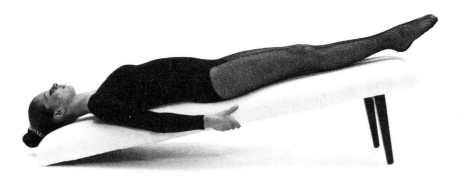

a

From Starting Position (a), flex both feet. **Breathe in** as you lift both legs up to vertical position, keeping knees as straight as possible (b).

Breathe out as you stretch both legs to your right (c) and slowly circle legs around to Starting Position (a). Relax.

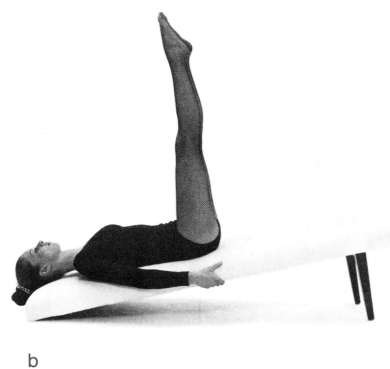

b

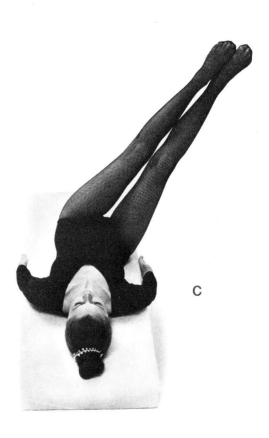

c

From Starting Position (a), flex both feet. **Breathe in** as you lift both legs up to a vertical position, keeping knees as straight as possible (d).

Breathe out as you stretch both legs to your left (e) and slowly circle legs around to Starting Position (a). Relax.

Alternate movements from right to left and from left to right.

Repeat circles in both directions five times.

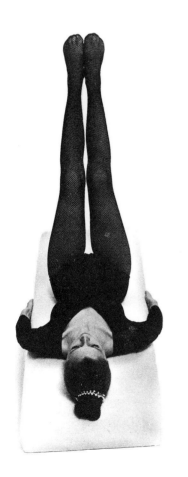

d

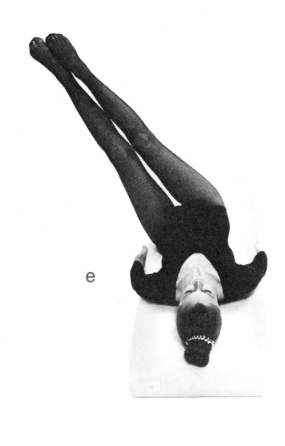

e

You have just completed the basic Body Rhythms performed on the slantboard. This is the most satisfactory and comfortable way to practice these Body Rhythms. The slant encourages circulation to the upper part of the body faster than when you are lying on a flat surface. If you have weak muscles in the abdomen and lower back, the slant position will speed up your progress and will prevent you from straining the muscles in the lumbar region.

I cannot overemphasize the importance of keeping your lower back flat on the slantboard throughout the entire Body Rhythms routine. Never let the lower back sway in. Swayback causes weakness in the lumbar and abdominal area and is the cause of bad posture. Body Rhythms will correct this weakness and improve posture, which is the foundation for good health and long lasting beauty.

To make it easy for you to get off the slantboard, bring both knees up to your chest. Turn on your side, place right hand on floor for support, and bring your knees down at the same time.

body rhythms for a lovely, youthful neckline (7-10)

To correct or prevent sagging neck muscles, double chin, dowager's hump, and to release tension at back of neck perform these rhythmic neck movements as slowly as possible. You will find them most relaxing. If you do them at night, you will sleep more soundly and wake up rested and refreshed.

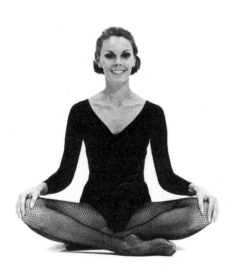

STARTING POSITION
Sit on floor, crosslegged, spine as straight as possible, shoulders relaxed, abdomen pulled in. Hands placed on knees.

body rhythm 7
VERTICAL NECK STRETCH

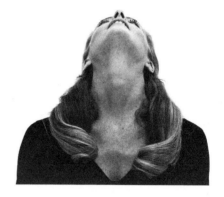

c

From Starting Position (a), **breathe in** as you slowly lower head forward, chin into chest (b).

Breathe out, return to Starting Position.

Breathe in, stretch head way back with chin up (c).

Breathe out, return to Starting Position. Relax.

Repeat five times in both directions.

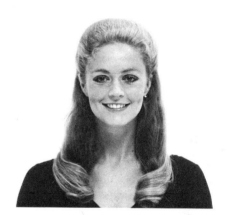

a

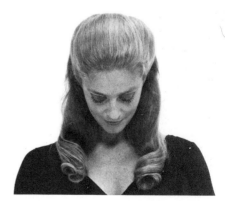

b

From Starting Position (a), **breathe in**, stretch head to right (b).

Breathe out, return to Starting Position.

Breathe in, stretch head to left (c).

Breathe out, return to Starting Position. Relax.

Repeat five times in both directions.

body rhythm 8
HORIZONTAL NECK STRETCH

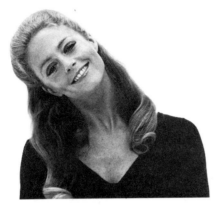

b

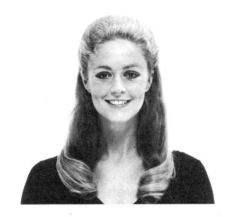

a

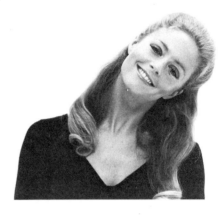

c

body rhythm 9
CHIN/NECK STRETCH

From Staring Position (a), stretch head way back, chin up (b).

Breathe in, stretch chin as far right as possible, keeping chin up all the time (c).

Breathe out, stretch chin as far left as possible, keeping chin up (d).

Alternate from right to left five times.

Return to center (b). Lower to Starting Position (a).

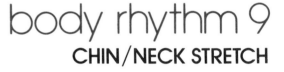

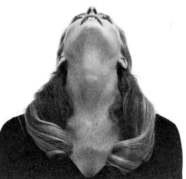

b

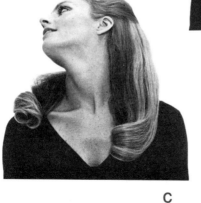

c

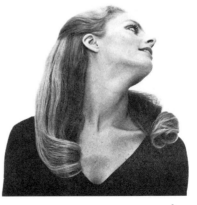

d

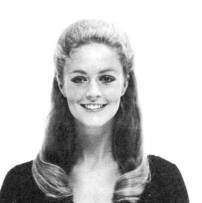

a

51

From Starting Position (a), drop head forward (b).

Breathe in, stretch head sideways to right and circle head way back (c, d, e) toward center with chin up (f).

Breathe out, circle head toward left, way down (g, h, i), back to (b) and up to center (a).

Reverse circle, moving from left to right.

Alternate these circle movements from right to left and left to right. Relax after you complete each circle.

Repeat five times.

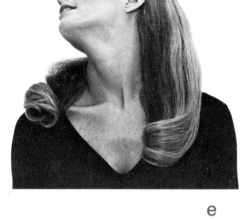

e

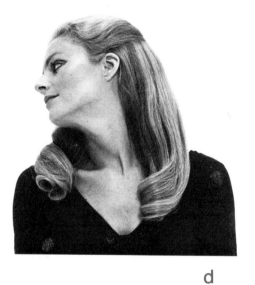

d

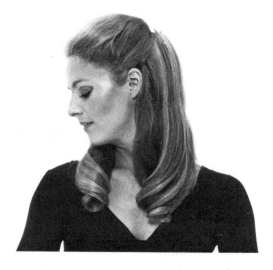

c

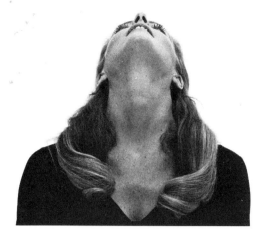

f

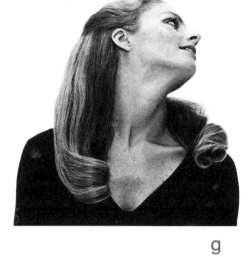

g

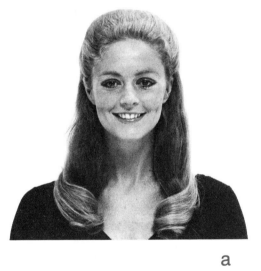

a

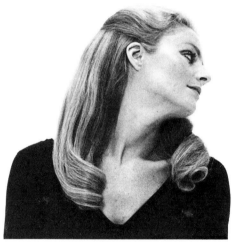

h

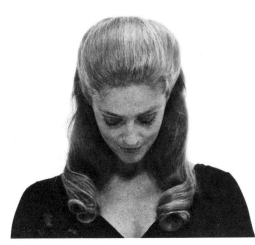

b

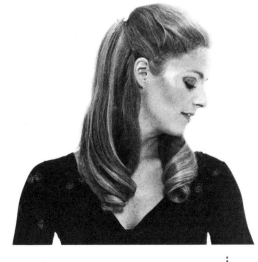

i

body rhythms for upper arms and shoulders (11-15)

To strengthen weak muscles in shoulders, improve bustline, firm and strengthen muscles in upper arms

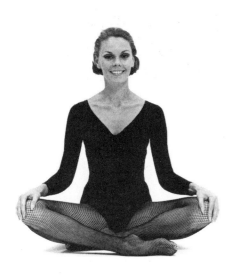

STARTING POSITION

Sit on floor, crosslegged, spine as straight as possible, shoulders relaxed and abdomen pulled in. Hands placed on knees.

body rhythm 11
ARM STRETCH I

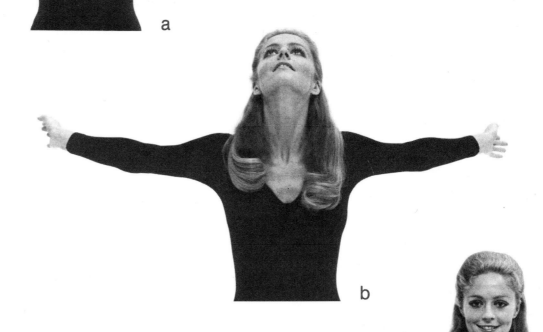

From Starting Position, bring arms forward at shoulder level, palms touching (a).

Breathe in, stretch both arms out sideways with hands flexed way back, stretching head back at the same time (b). Bounce arms back and forth three times at shoulder level.

a

b

Breathe out, bring arms back to center, palms touching (c). Relax.

Repeat five times.

c

Place hands on shoulders with elbows touching the sides of the body (a).

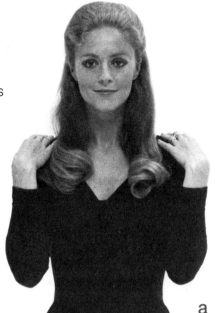

a

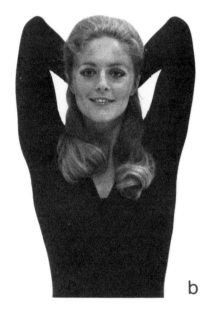

b

Breathe in, bring both elbows forward and up (b).

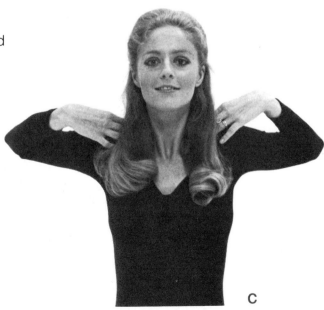

c

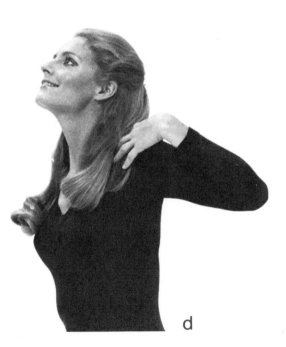

d

Breathe out, circle elbows to shoulder level (c) and down (d) to Starting Position. Relax.

Repeat five times.

55

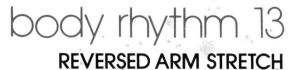

body rhythm 13
REVERSED ARM STRETCH

From Starting Position, bring arms forward at shoulder level, palms touching (a).

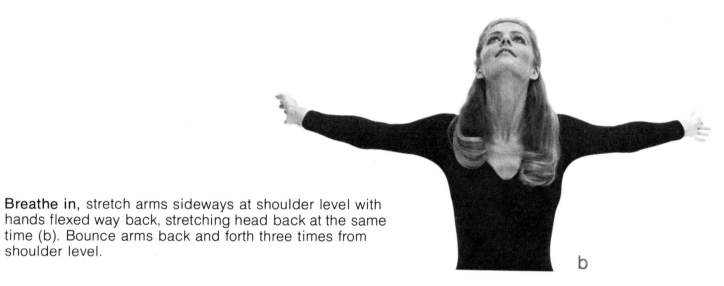

a

Breathe in, stretch arms sideways at shoulder level with hands flexed way back, stretching head back at the same time (b). Bounce arms back and forth three times from shoulder level.

b

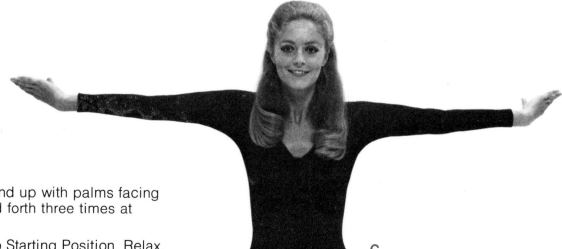

Breathe out, turn hands out and up with palms facing up (c). Bounce arms back and forth three times at shoulder level.

Alternate five times. Return to Starting Position. Relax.

c

56

body rhythm 14
CLASPED HAND STRETCH

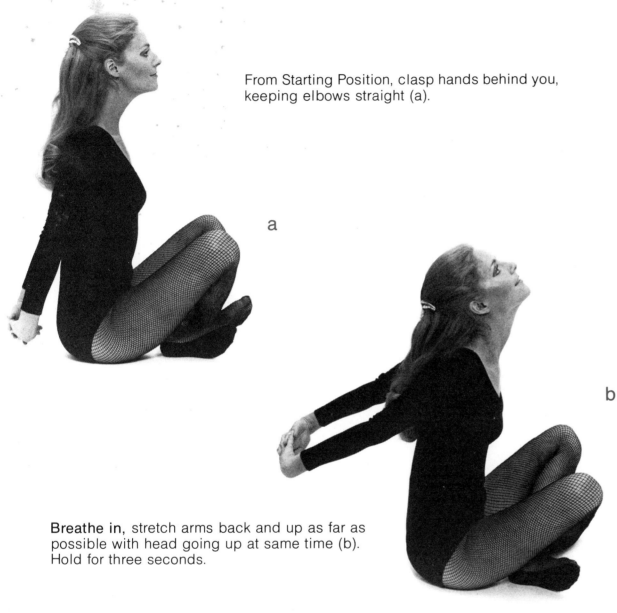

a

From Starting Position, clasp hands behind you, keeping elbows straight (a).

b

Breathe in, stretch arms back and up as far as possible with head going up at same time (b). Hold for three seconds.

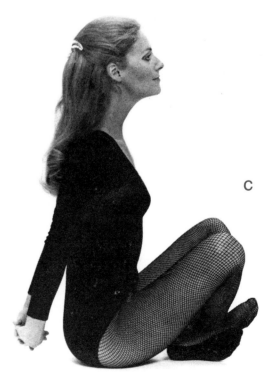

c

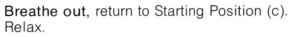

Breathe out, return to Starting Position (c). Relax.

Repeat five times.

57

From Starting Position, **breathe in,** stretch arms overhead, elbows straight, back of hands touching (a).

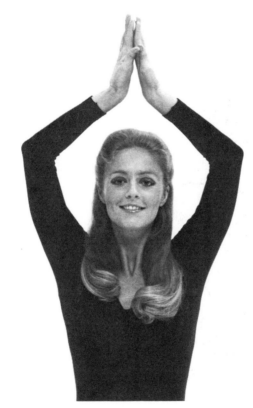

a

b

Breathe out, lower arms by bending elbows (b), and place back of hands on shoulders with elbows at shoulder level (c).

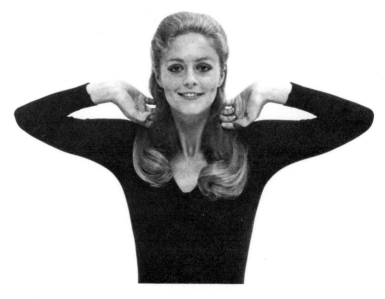

c

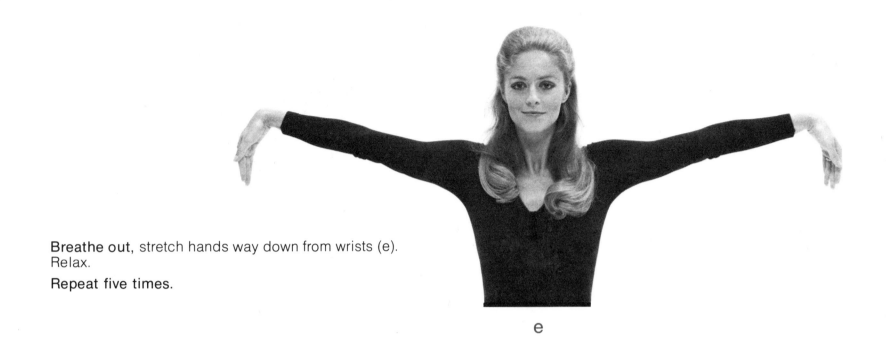

Breathe out, stretch hands way down from wrists (e). Relax.

Repeat five times.

e

Breathe in, stretch arms way out, still at shoulder level with hands flexed upward (d).

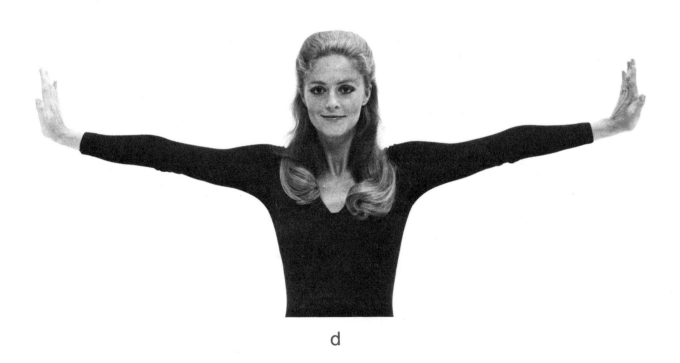

d

body rhythms for weak muscles

in lower back (16-18)

To stretch and strengthen muscles in lower back, improve posture, relieve tension and fatigue.

BODY RHYTHMS 16 and 17 are difficult movements that must be practiced with great care. Begin by stretching your entire torso forward without straining, moving from hip joints. With daily practice the muscles in your lower back will become stronger and more elastic, and you will be able to bend your torso forward and sideways with ease.

Remember to coordinate breathing with each movement. This will prevent you from tiring and will ensure slow, rhythmic movements at all times.

STARTING POSITION
Sit on floor, spine as straight as possible, shoulders relaxed, abdomen pulled in, legs stretched wide apart, knees straight.

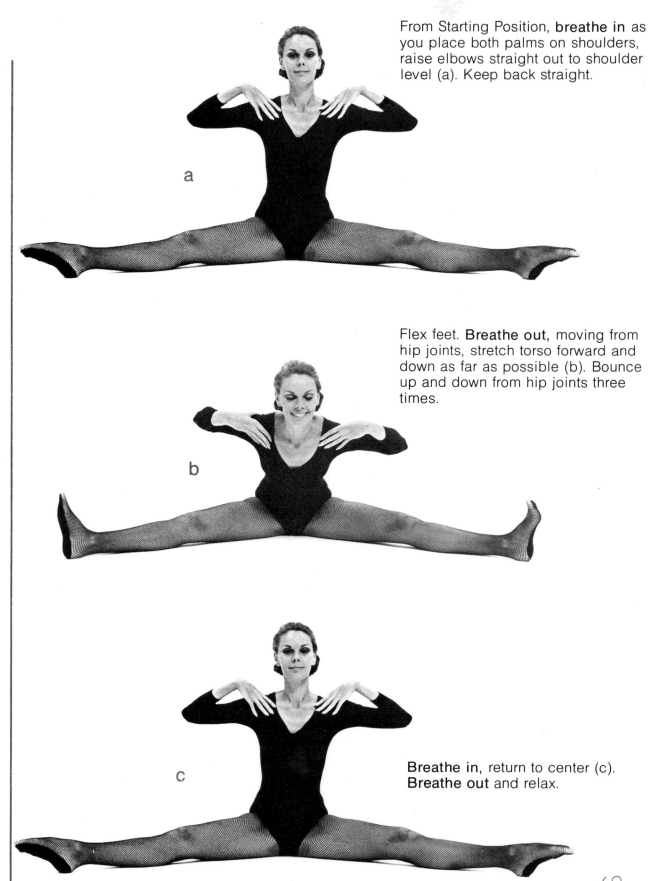

From Starting Position, **breathe in** as you place both palms on shoulders, raise elbows straight out to shoulder level (a). Keep back straight.

Flex feet. **Breathe out**, moving from hip joints, stretch torso forward and down as far as possible (b). Bounce up and down from hip joints three times.

Breathe in, return to center (c). **Breathe out** and relax.

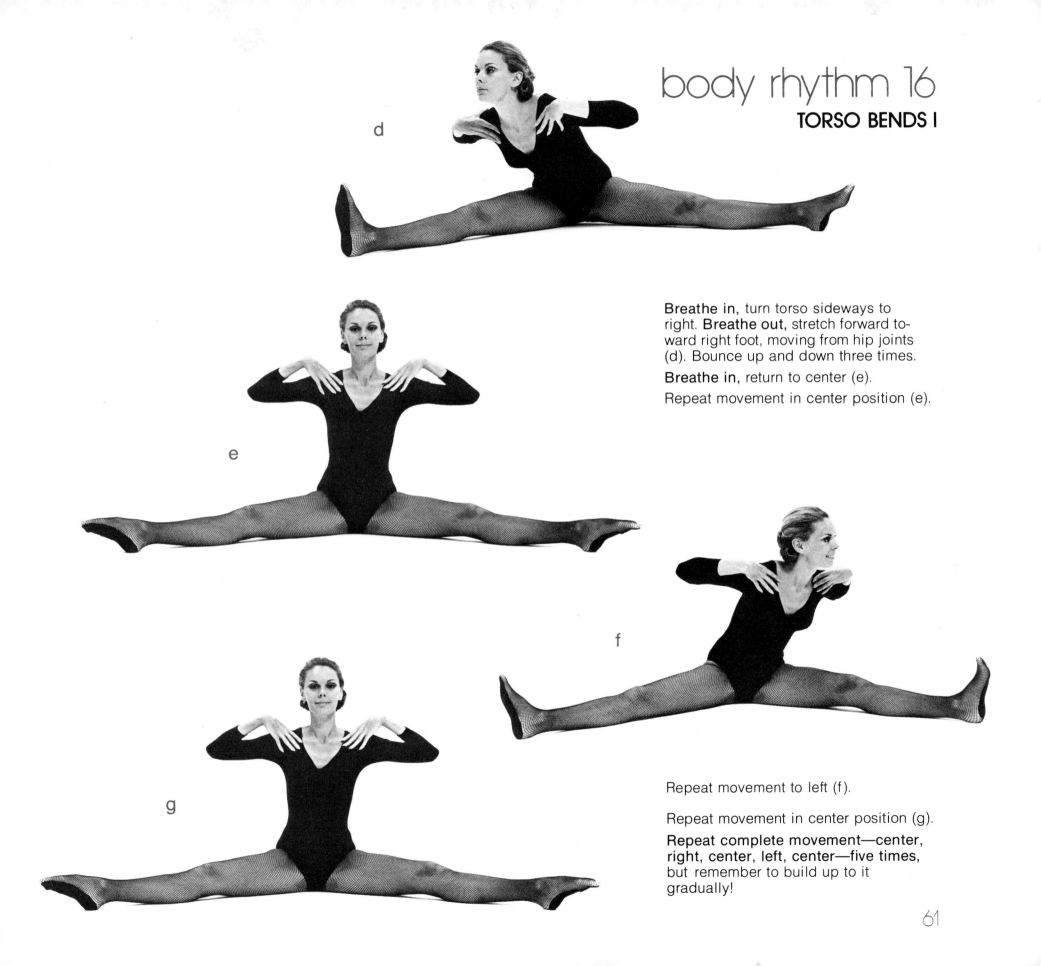

d

Breathe in, turn torso sideways to right. Breathe out, stretch forward toward right foot, moving from hip joints (d). Bounce up and down three times.

Breathe in, return to center (e).

Repeat movement in center position (e).

e

f

g

Repeat movement to left (f).

Repeat movement in center position (g).

Repeat complete movement—center, right, center, left, center—five times, but remember to build up to it gradually!

61

body rhythm 17
TORSO BENDS II

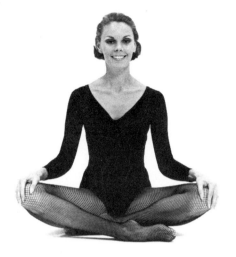

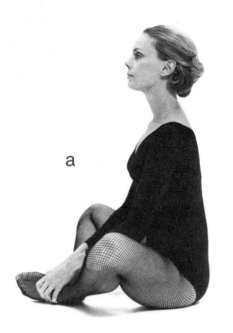

a

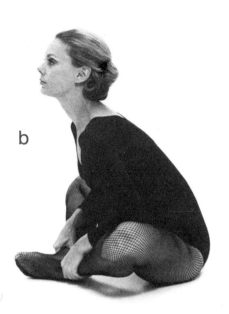

b

STARTING POSITION

Sit on floor, crosslegged, spine as straight as possible, shoulders relaxed, abdomen pulled in. Place hands on knees.

From Starting Position, **breathe in,** bend both knees and bring feet in, grasping ankles with both hands (a).

Breathe out, bring torso forward and down as far as possible, moving from hip joints (b). Bounce up and down three times.

Breathe in, return to (a). Relax.

Repeat five times.

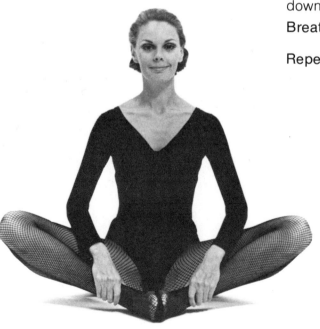

a

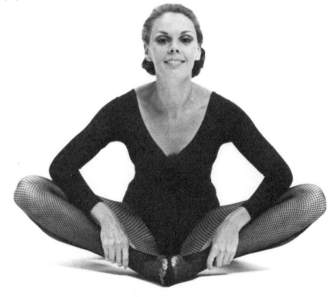

b

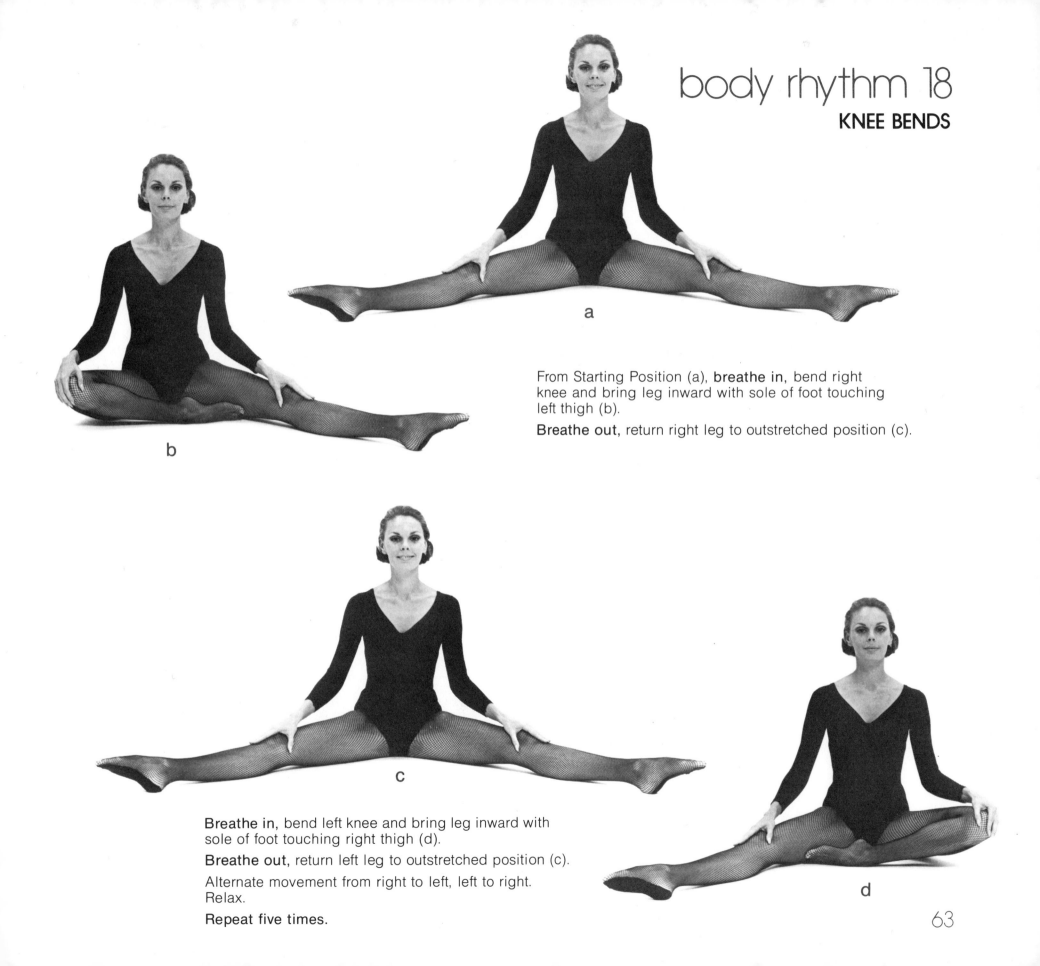

body rhythm 18
KNEE BENDS

From Starting Position (a), **breathe in,** bend right knee and bring leg inward with sole of foot touching left thigh (b).

Breathe out, return right leg to outstretched position (c).

a

b

c

Breathe in, bend left knee and bring leg inward with sole of foot touching right thigh (d).

Breathe out, return left leg to outstretched position (c).

Alternate movement from right to left, left to right. Relax.

Repeat five times.

d

BODY ROLLS

body rhythms for hips, thighs,

calves and ankles (19-21)

Triple-action rhythmic movements to slim, reshape and strengthen hips, thighs, calves and ankles

If space is available, do five Rolls across room in one direction. Reverse and return to starting place. If space is limited, do only two or three Rolls.

Remember:

1. Keep abdomen pulled in.
2. Keep back straight.
3. Keep buttocks firm.

STARTING POSITION

Lie on floor in a half-reclining position, knees straight, toes pointed. Place palms down and forward behind torso. Raise feet 12 inches off floor (a).

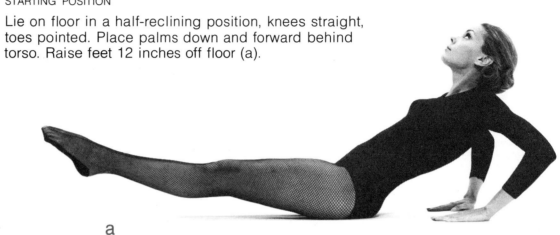

a

Breathe in, roll over onto left hip and thigh (b).

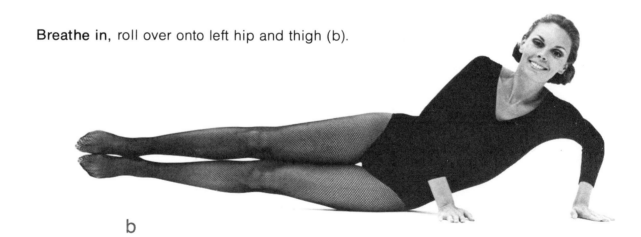

b

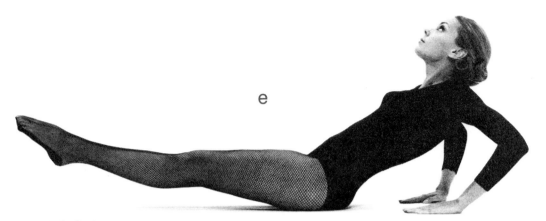

e

Breathe out and return to Starting Position (e). Relax.
Repeat same movement in the opposite direction.
Repeat five times.

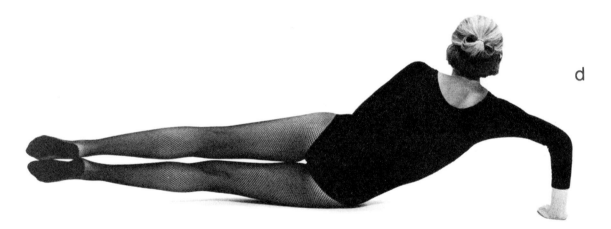

d

Breathe in, roll over onto right hip and thigh (d).

Breathe out, roll over onto abdomen, resting on hips and
thighs (c).

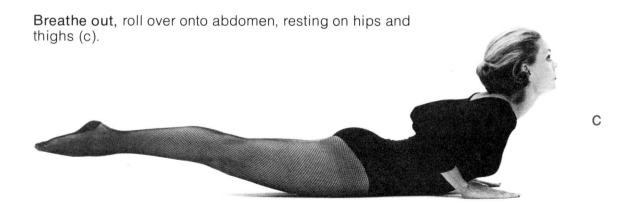

c

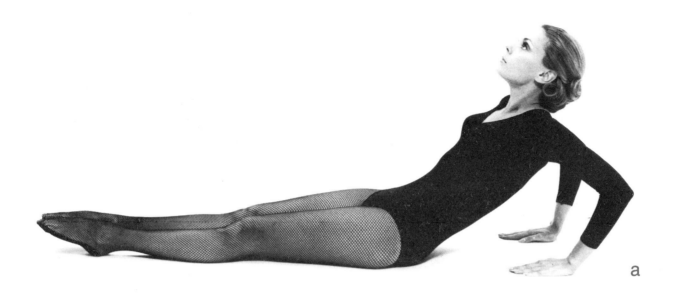

a

STARTING POSITION

Lie on floor in a half-reclining position, knees straight, heels flat on floor, toes pointed. Place palms down, pointing forward behind torso (a).

b

Breathe in, bend both knees toward chest, chin up (b).

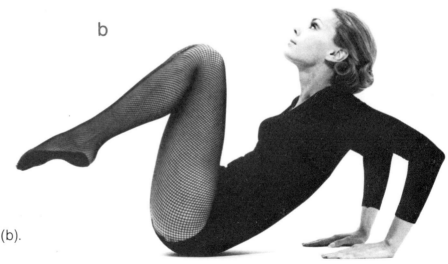

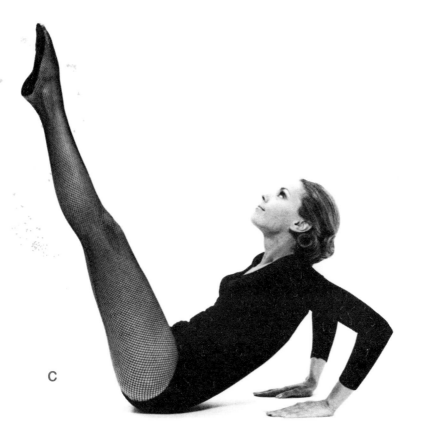

c

Breathe out, stretch both legs way up, knees straight, toes pointed (c).

Breathe in, flex both feet (d).

Breathe out, bring both legs slowly down to Starting Position (a). Relax.

Repeat five times.

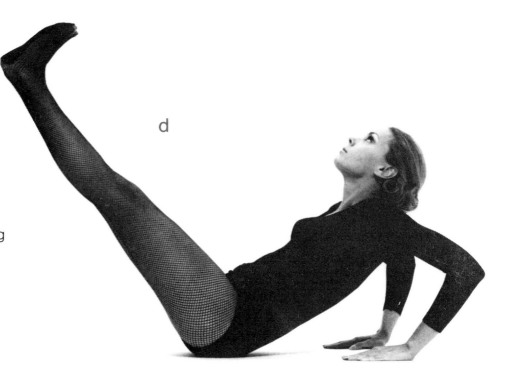

d

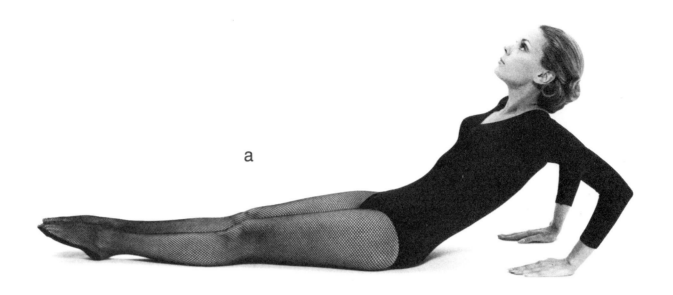

a

From Starting Position (a), lift right side of body and roll torso over onto left hip and thigh. Place palms on floor, knees straight, toes pointed (b).

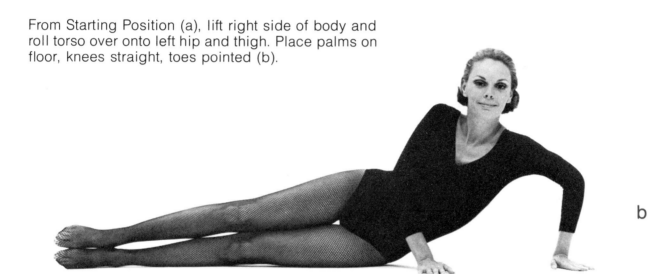

b

Breathe in, bend right knee toward shoulder (c).

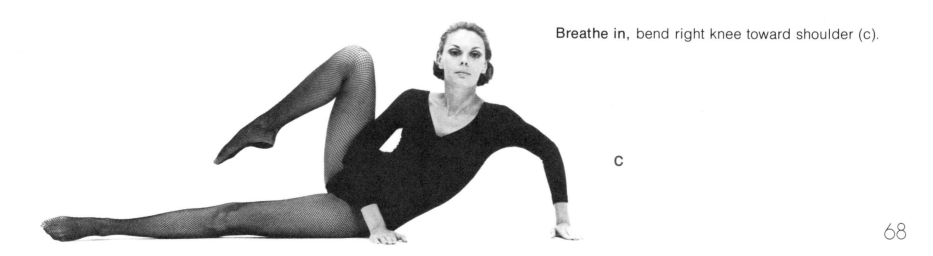

c

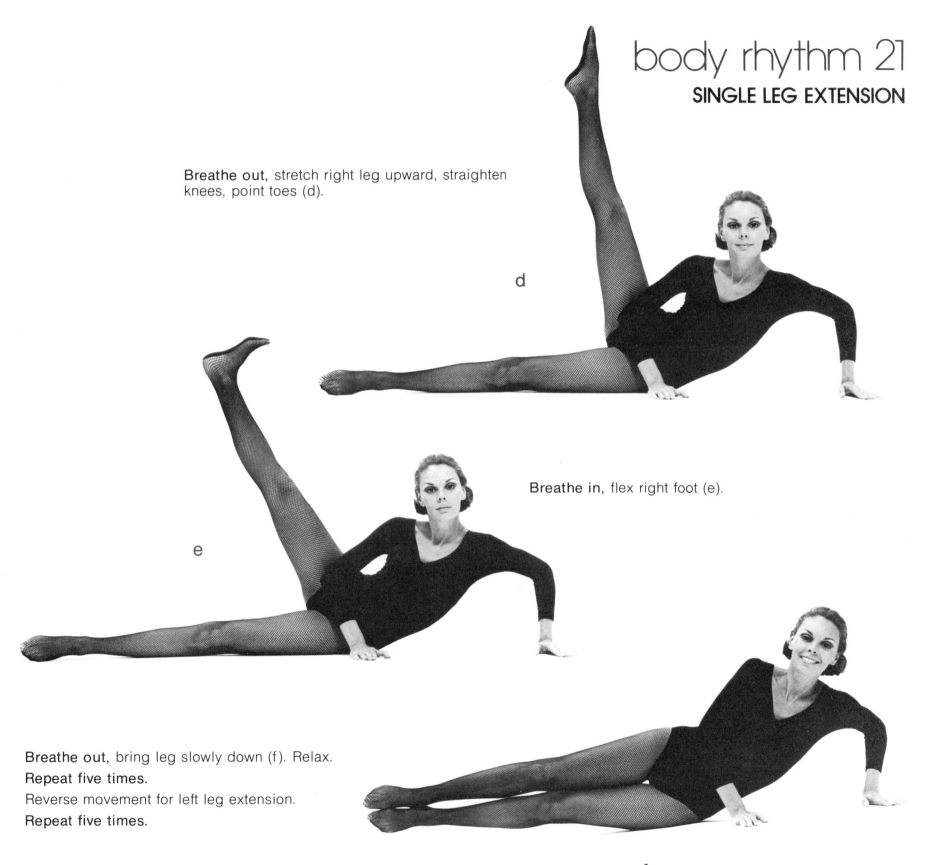

Breathe out, stretch right leg upward, straighten knees, point toes (d).

d

Breathe in, flex right foot (e).

e

Breathe out, bring leg slowly down (f). Relax.
Repeat five times.
Reverse movement for left leg extension.
Repeat five times.

f

69

body rhythms for
overall flexibility and grace
of movement (22-28)

Rhythmic movements to reshape and firm arms, to strengthen upper shoulders and lower back.

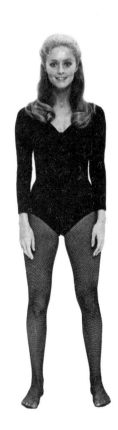

Stand erect with feet pointing forward about 10 inches apart, arms at sides, elbows straight.

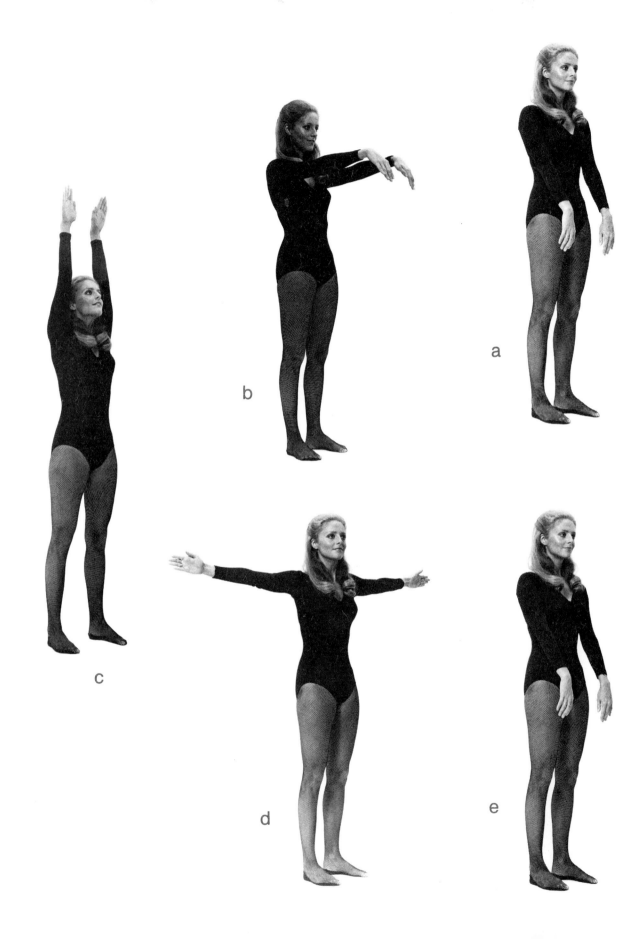

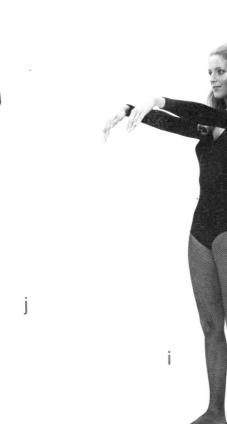

body rhythm 22
ARM CIRCLES I

Breathe in, stretch arms forward and way up (a, b, c).

Breathe out, bring arms way back and down to Starting Position (d, e). Relax.

Repeat movement in opposite direction with palms facing forward.

Breathe in, stretch both arms way back and up (f, g, h).

Breathe out, lower arms forward and down to Starting Position (i, j). Relax.

Repeat complete movement five times.

j

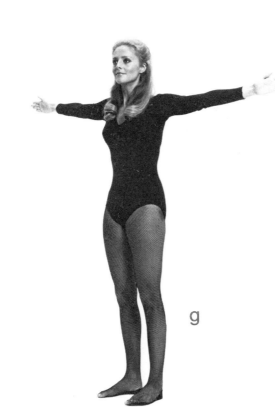

i

f

g

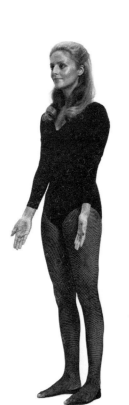

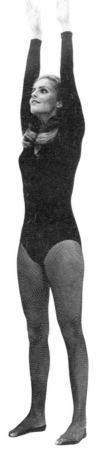

h

Clench hands into tight fists and turn fists out, stretching from wrists (a).

Breathe in, bring both arms forward and up (b, c).

Breathe out, stretch arms way back and down (d, e, f). Relax.

Repeat movement in opposite direction.

Breathe in, stretch both arms way back and up (g, h, i, j).

Breathe out, bring both arms forward and down (k, l). Relax.

Do not release clenched fists throughout circles.

Repeat complete movement five times.

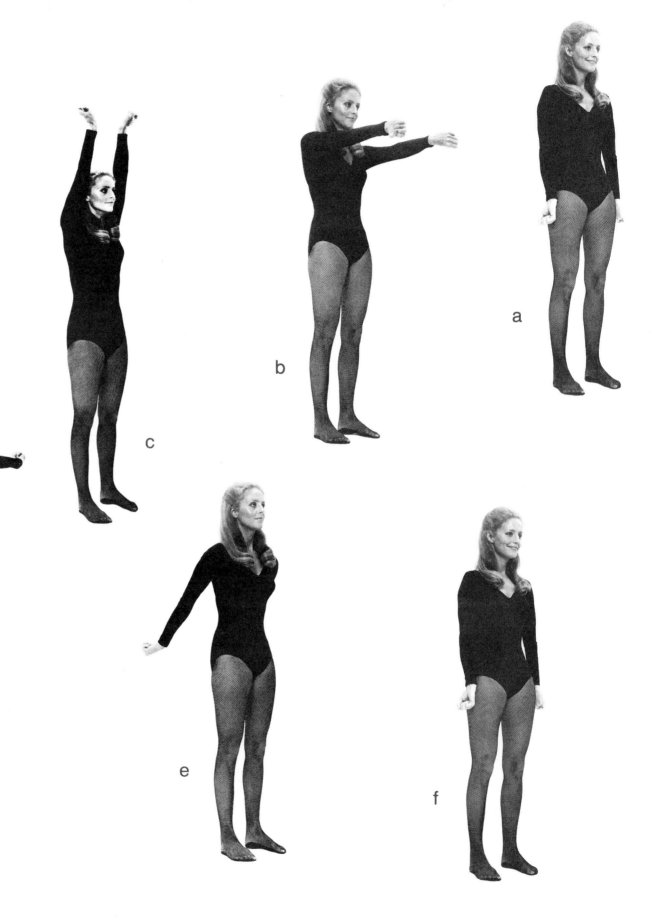

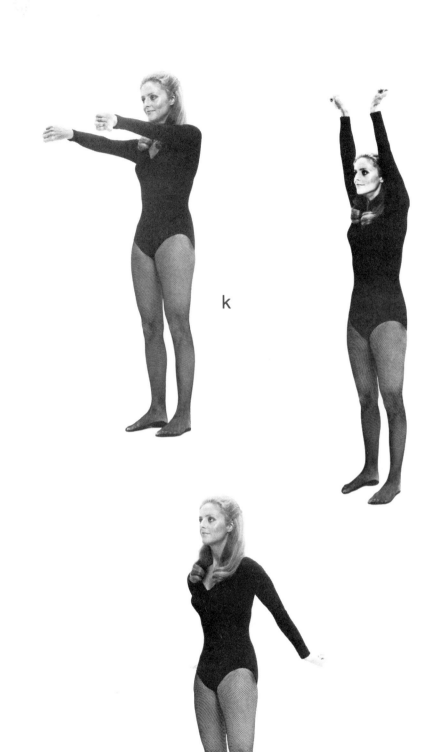

l

k

j

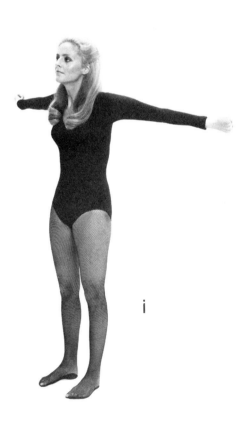

g

h

i

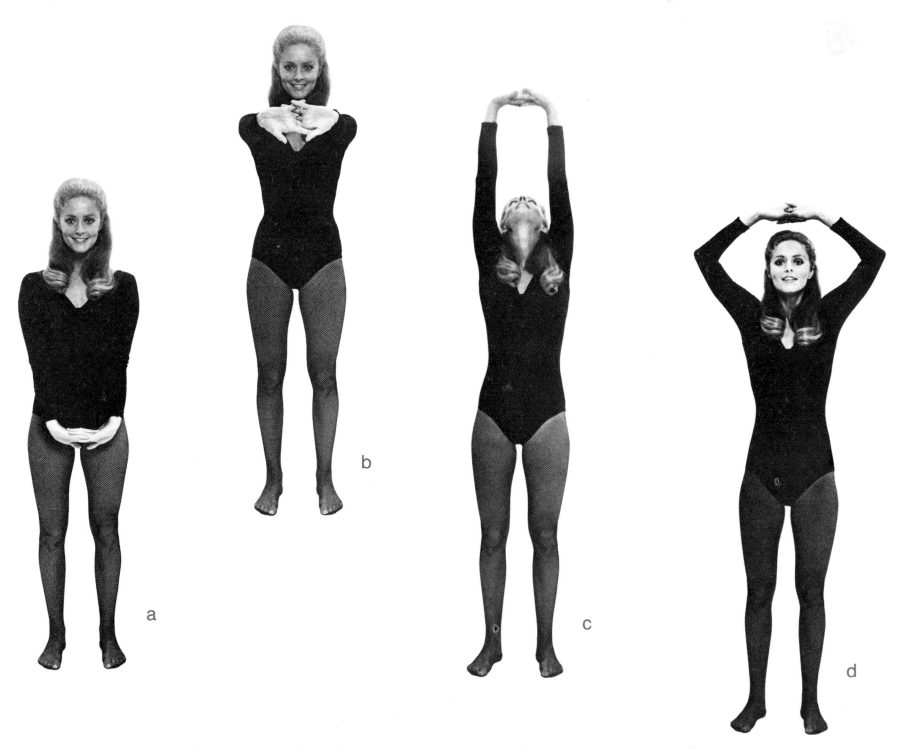

Clasp hands in front of you (a). **Breathe in,** stretch arms forward and above head with palms up, elbows straight (b, c).

Breathe out, lower arms over head by bending elbows (d).

Breathe in, sway body to right from waistline and bounce three times (e).

Breathe out, return to upright position (f). **Breathe in,** stretch arms above head (c). **Breathe out,** lower arms over head (d).

Breathe in, sway body to left from waistline (g) and bounce three times.

Breathe out, return to upright position (f). **Breathe in,** stretch arms above head (c). **Breathe out,** lower arms over head (d). Relax.

Repeat five times in both directions.

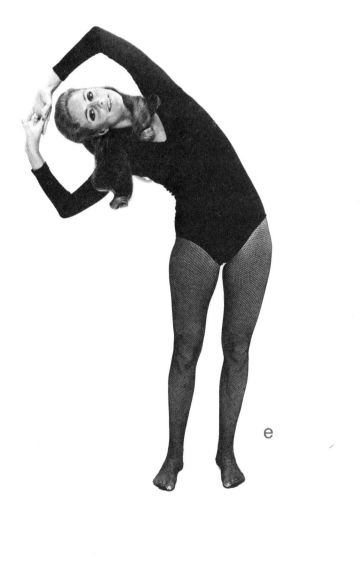

e

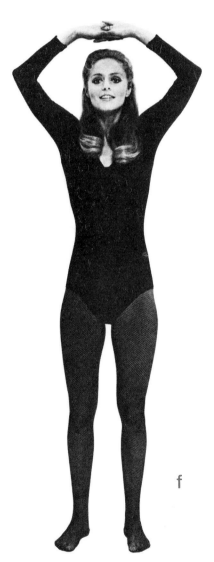

f

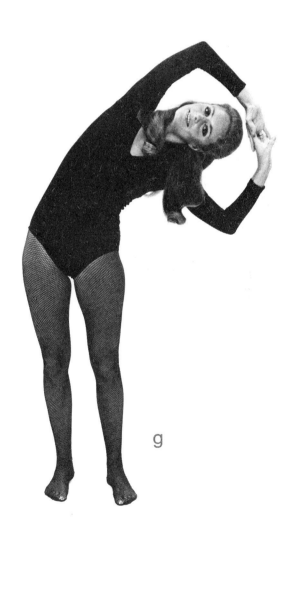

g

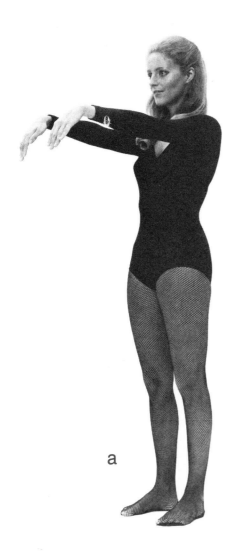

a

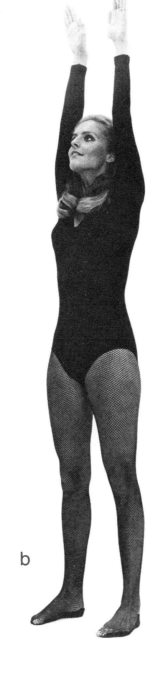

b

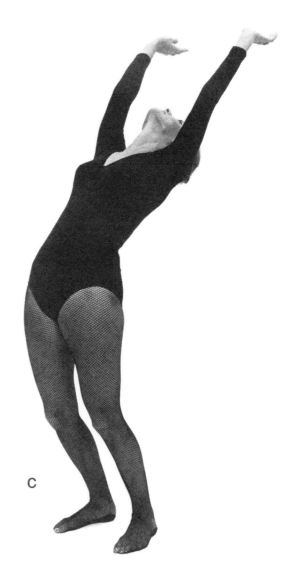

c

From Starting Position, **breathe in,**
raise both arms forward and way up
(a, b).

Breathe out, sway torso way back (c),
stretching from thighs. Bounce back
and forth three times.

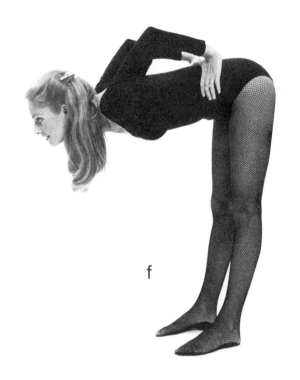

f

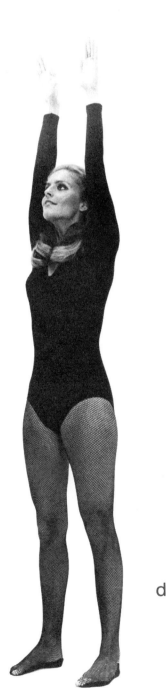

d

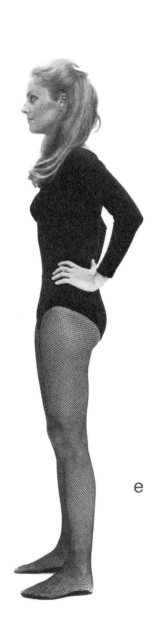

e

Breathe in, return to upright position (d), placing hands at waistline (e).

Breathe out, bend torso forward and down moving from hip joints (f).

Keep back as straight as possible. Bounce three times up and down from hip joints. Return to (e).

Relax.

Return to upright position (a, b) and **repeat movement five times.**

Place hands at waistline (a).

Breathe in, bend torso forward and down, moving from hip joints (b).

Breathe out and bounce up and down from hip joints three times.

Breathe in, stretch torso sideways to right, circling way up to center, stretching head way back (c, d, e).

Breathe out, stretch torso sideways to left circling way down, back to center (f, g, h). Bounce up and down three times from hip joints.

Repeat entire circle movement in opposite direction—toward left.

Repeat complete movement from right to left and left to right five times.

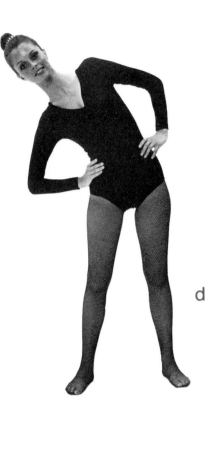

d

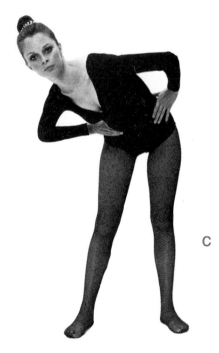

c

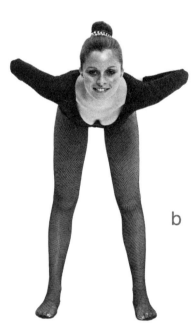

b

78

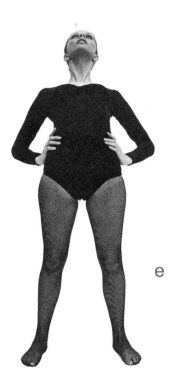

e

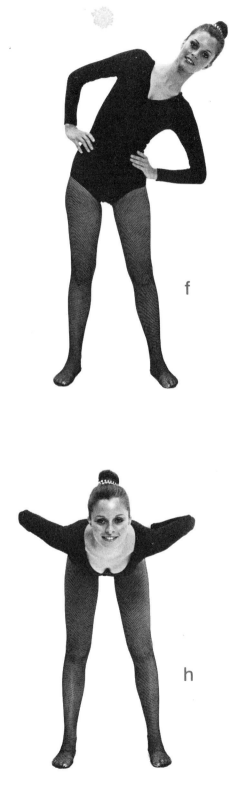

f

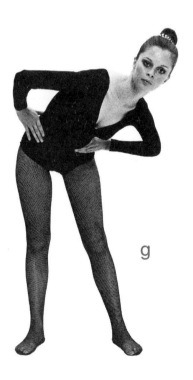

g

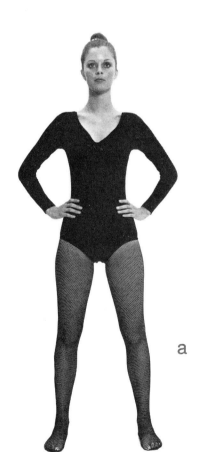

a

h

body rhythm 26

TORSO CIRCLES

79

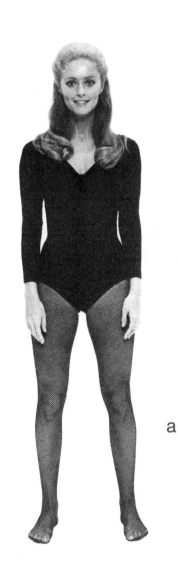

a

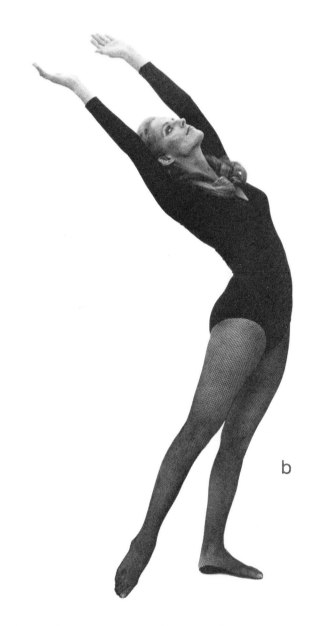

b

From Starting Position (a), **breathe in,** swing arms up and turn torso sideways to left.

Breathe out, lift right heel off floor, and bounce back and forth three times (b).

Breathe in, return to center (c), and turn torso sideways to right.

80

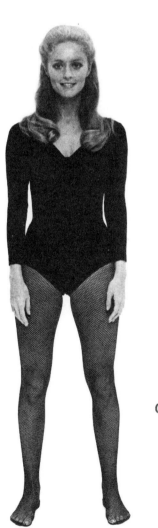

c

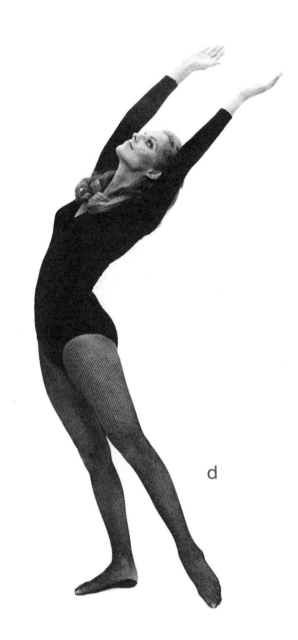

d

Breathe out, lift left heel off floor, and bounce back and forth three times (d).

Breathe in, return to Starting Position (a). Relax.

Repeat five times.

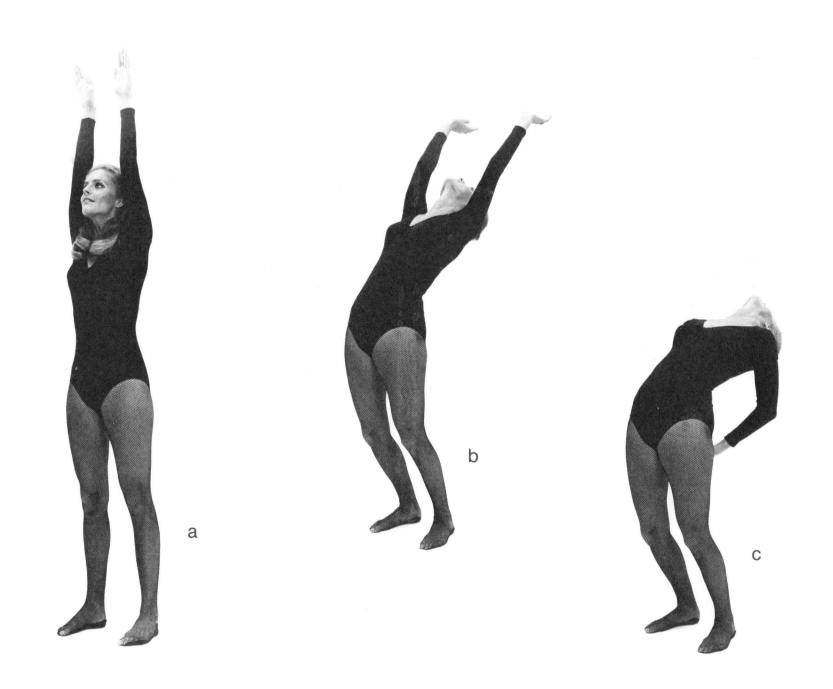

a

b

c

TORSO STRETCH II

From Starting Position, **breathe in,** raise both arms forward and way up (a).

Breathe out, sway torso way back, and bounce back and forth three times stretching from thighs (b).

Breathe in, clasping hands behind you (c), bring torso back to upright position.

Breathe out, bend torso forward and down with hands and arms stretching way up behind you (d, e). Bounce three times from hip joints.

Return to Starting Position. Relax.

Repeat five times.

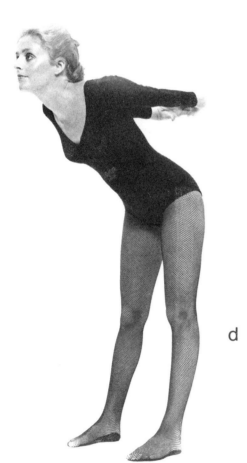

d

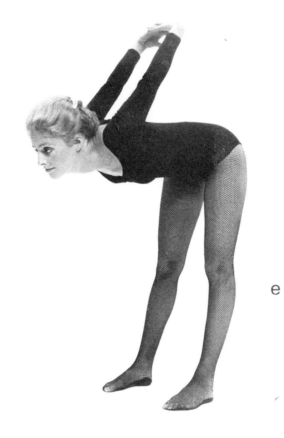

e

intermediate body rhythms

body rhythms for abdominal and spinal development (29-36)

The next eight Body Rhythms are intermediate movements, performed on the slantboard. Do not expect to accomplish them in a short time. Add only one intermediate movement at a time to the basic rhythms until your spinal column is strong enough to add the complete routine to your daily schedule.

Remember—what is important is thorough and proper execution of these rhythmic movements and not how quickly you accomplish them. Do not strain your body and do not hurry.

Do not attempt intermediate routines until Basic Body Rhythms are perfected.

STARTING POSITION
Lie flat on your back on slantboard, lower back pressing into board, arms at sides, hands holding onto board.

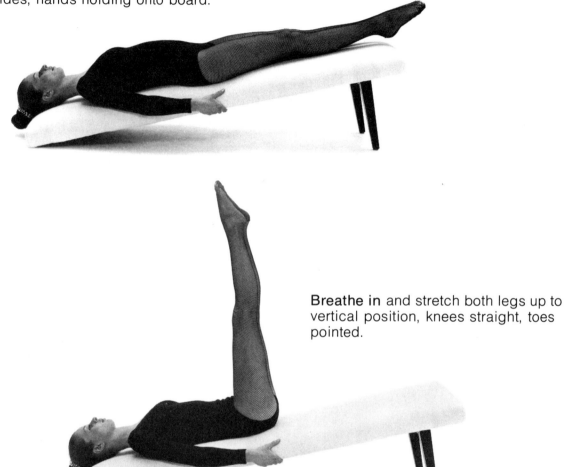

Breathe in and stretch both legs up to vertical position, knees straight, toes pointed.

Breathe out and slowly bring both legs down. Relax.

Repeat five times.

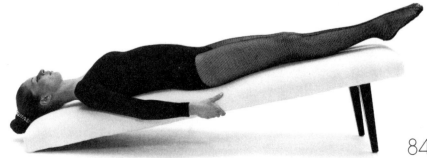

84

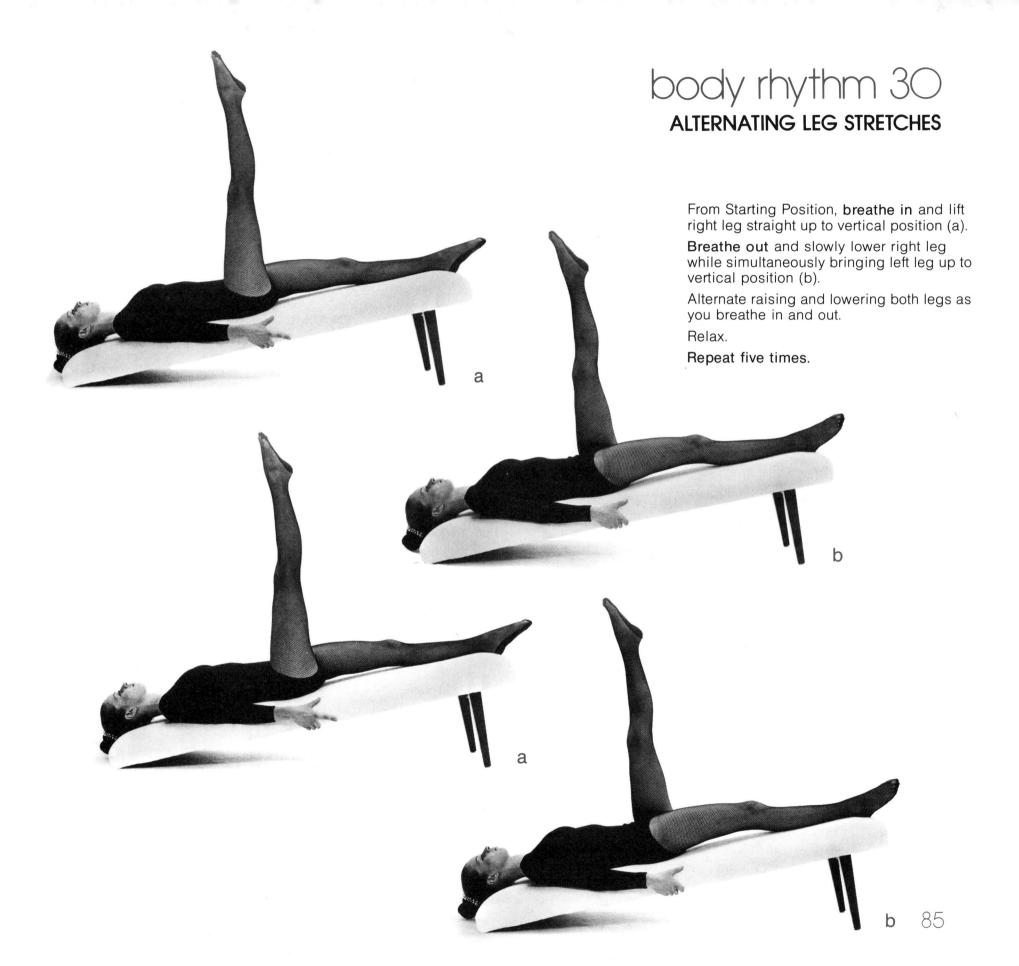

body rhythm 30
ALTERNATING LEG STRETCHES

From Starting Position, **breathe in** and lift right leg straight up to vertical position (a).

Breathe out and slowly lower right leg while simultaneously bringing left leg up to vertical position (b).

Alternate raising and lowering both legs as you breathe in and out.

Relax.

Repeat five times.

a

b

a

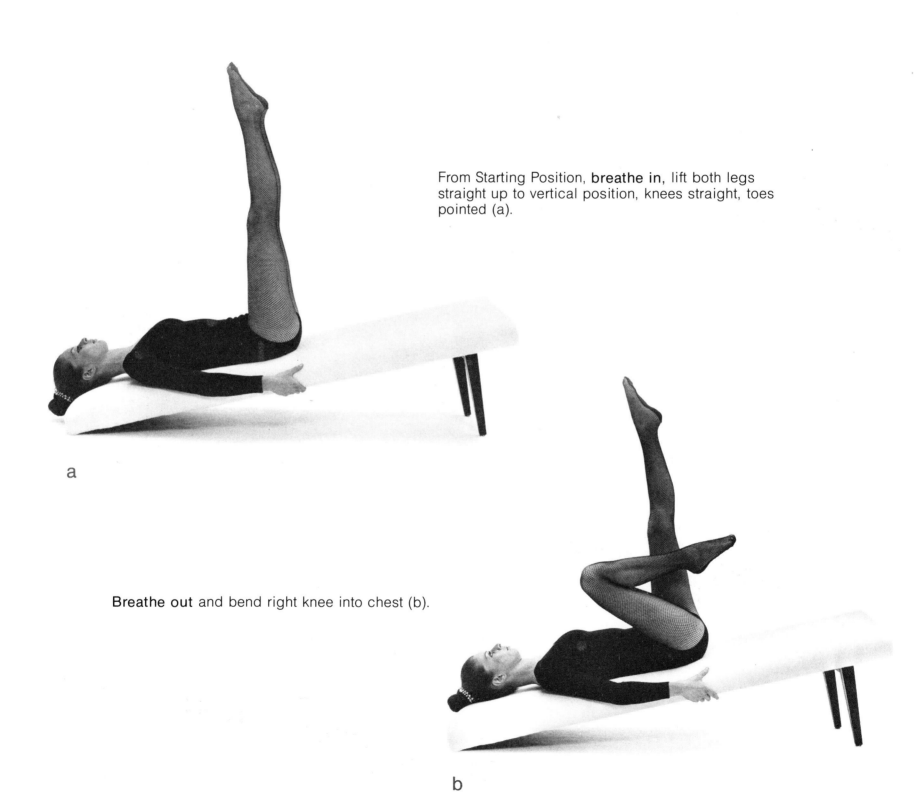

From Starting Position, **breathe in**, lift both legs straight up to vertical position, knees straight, toes pointed (a).

a

Breathe out and bend right knee into chest (b).

b

86

body rhythm 31
ALTERNATING KNEE BENDS

Breathe in, return left leg to vertical position (e).

Alternate knee bends from right to left and left to right, breathing in and out. Relax.

Repeat five times.

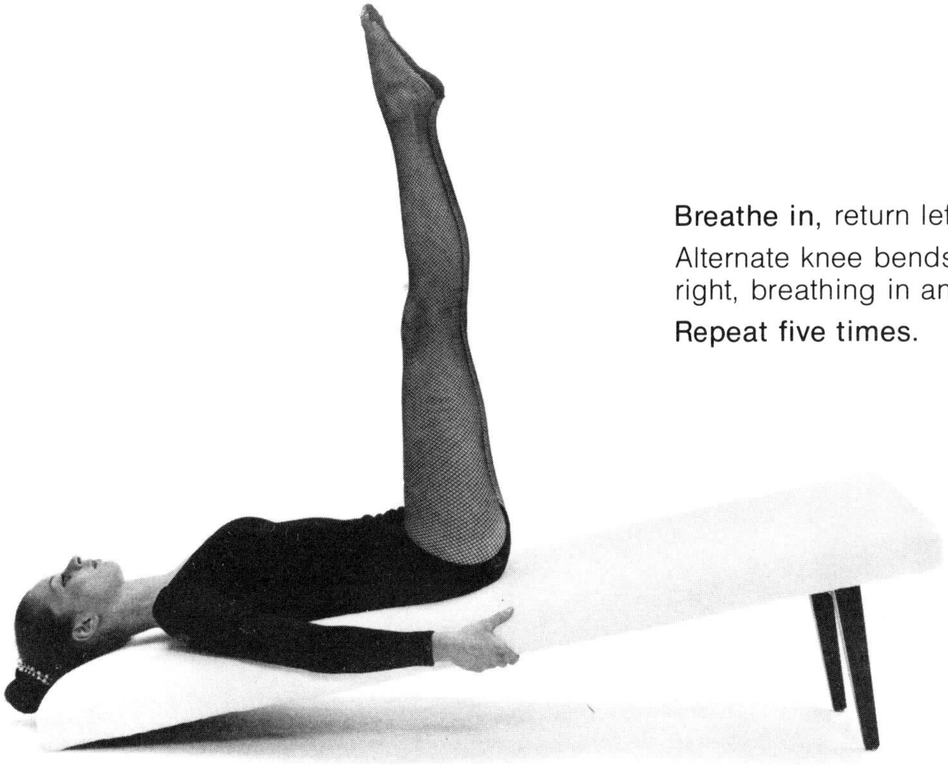

e

d

c

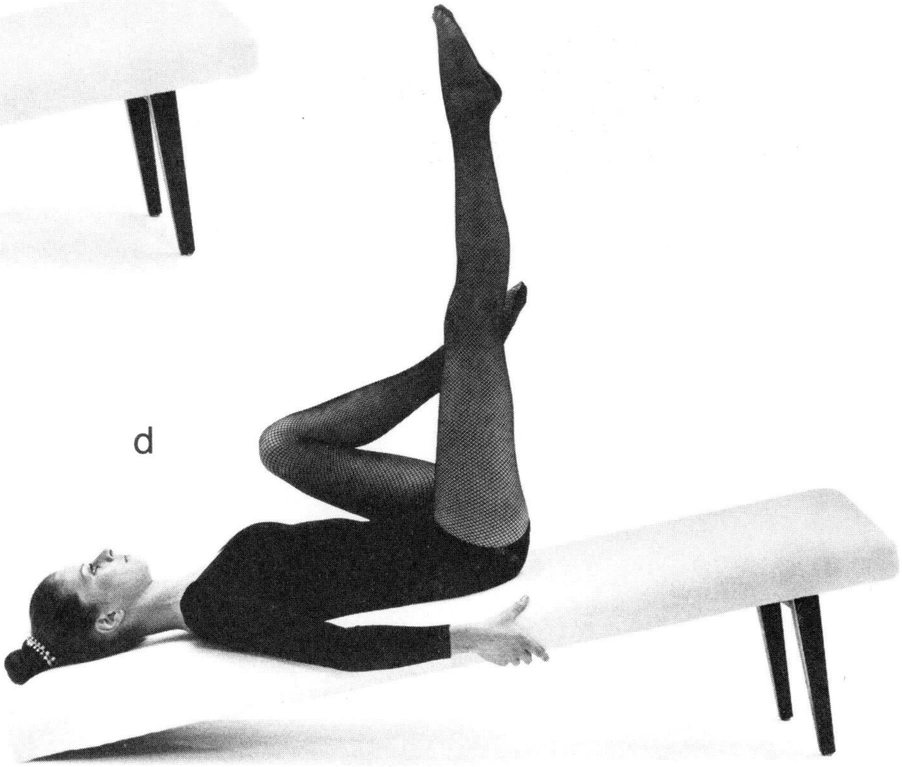

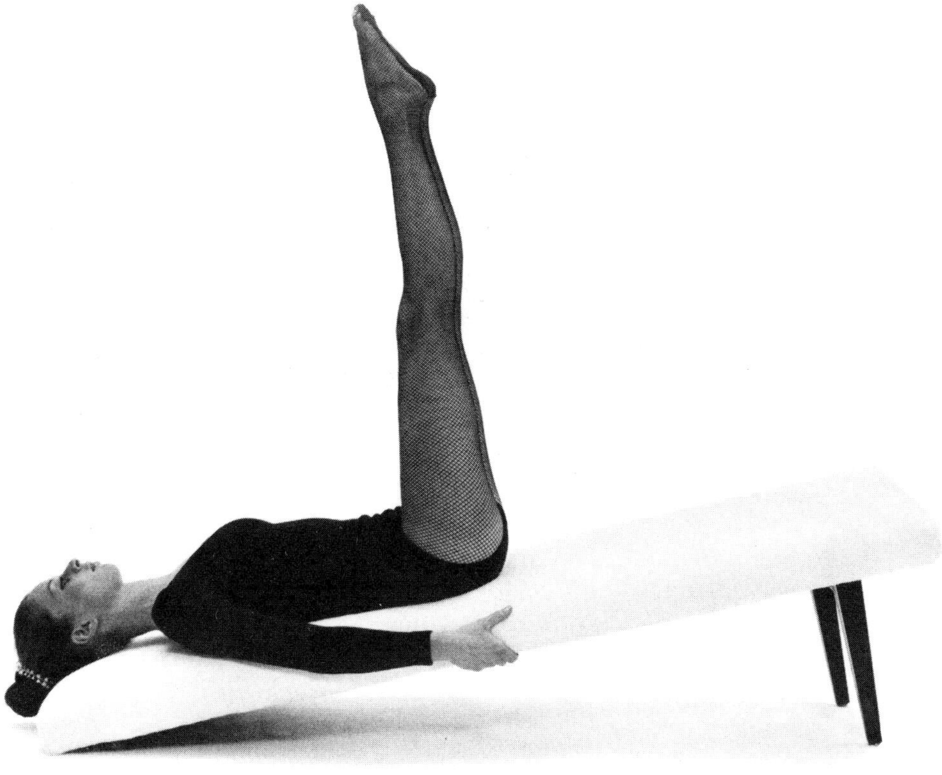

Breathe in, return right leg to vertical position (c).

Breathe out, bend left knee into chest (d).

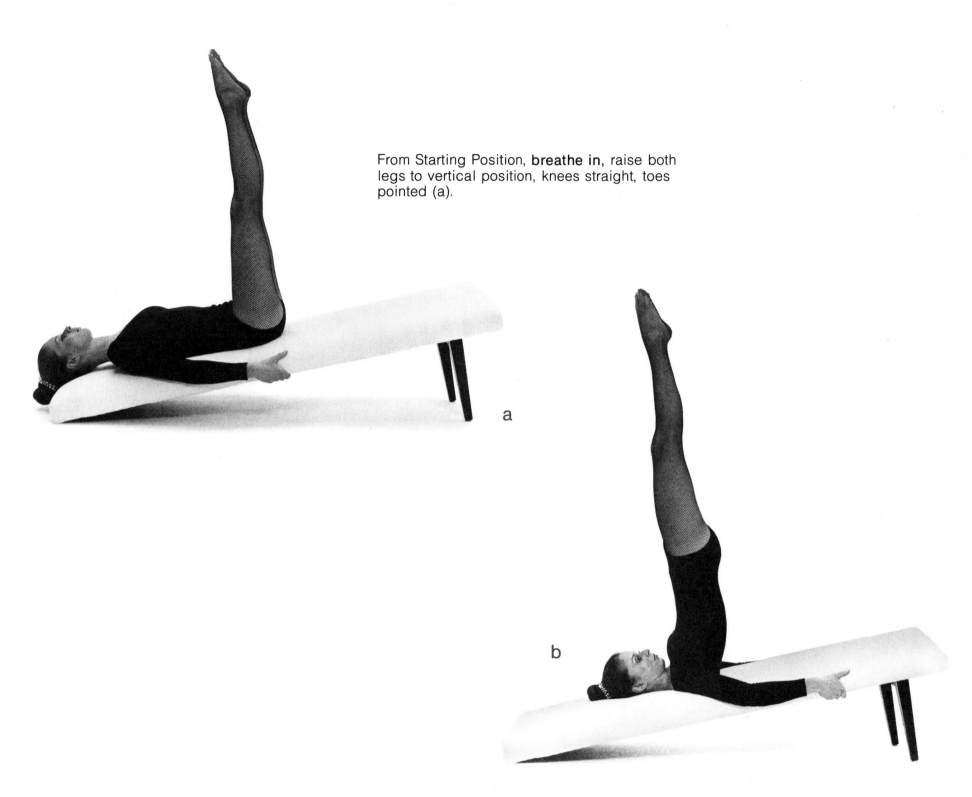

From Starting Position, **breathe in,** raise both legs to vertical position, knees straight, toes pointed (a).

a

b

Photos **b, c, d** show the body in the center of the board. This movement is actually performed with the head touching the end of the board as shown in the Starting Position.

Breathe out, lift entire torso off board, spine as straight as possible (b).

Breathe out. Bring torso slowly down to slantboard (e).

Return to Starting Position. Relax.

Repeat five times.

e

d

Breathe in, stretch both legs up to vertical position (d).

c

Moving from hip joints, lower both legs to a horizontal position over head (c).

89

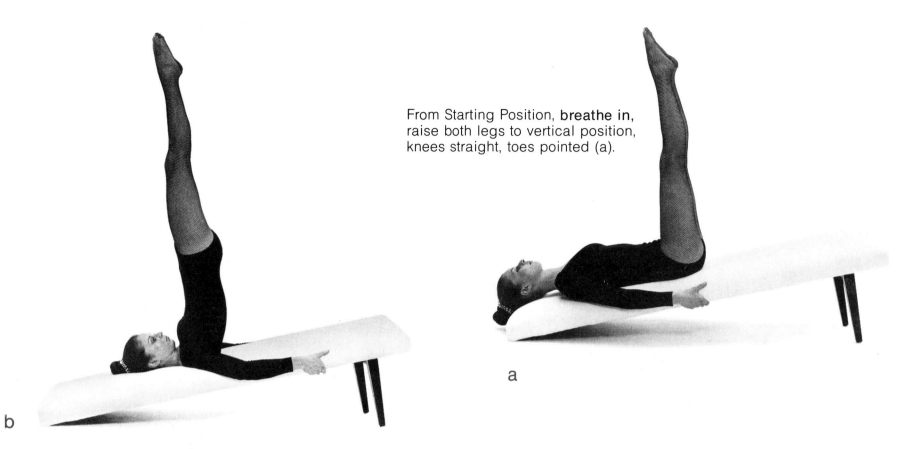

From Starting Position, **breathe in,** raise both legs to vertical position, knees straight, toes pointed (a).

Breathe out, lift entire torso off board, spine as straight as possible (b).

Moving from hip joints, lower both legs to horizontal position over head (c).

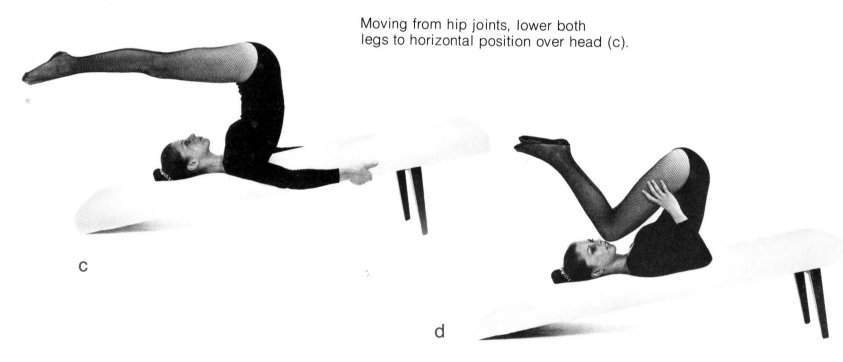

Breathe in, bend both knees and bring them into chest keeping torso off the board (d).

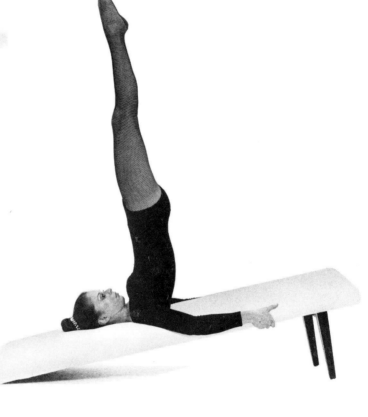

g

Breathe in, stretch both legs up to
vertical position (f). **Breathe out.**
Bring torso slowly down to slantboard (g).

Return to Starting Position. Relax.

Repeat five times.

f

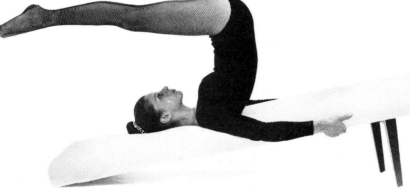

Breathe out, stretch legs back to
horizontal position (e).

e

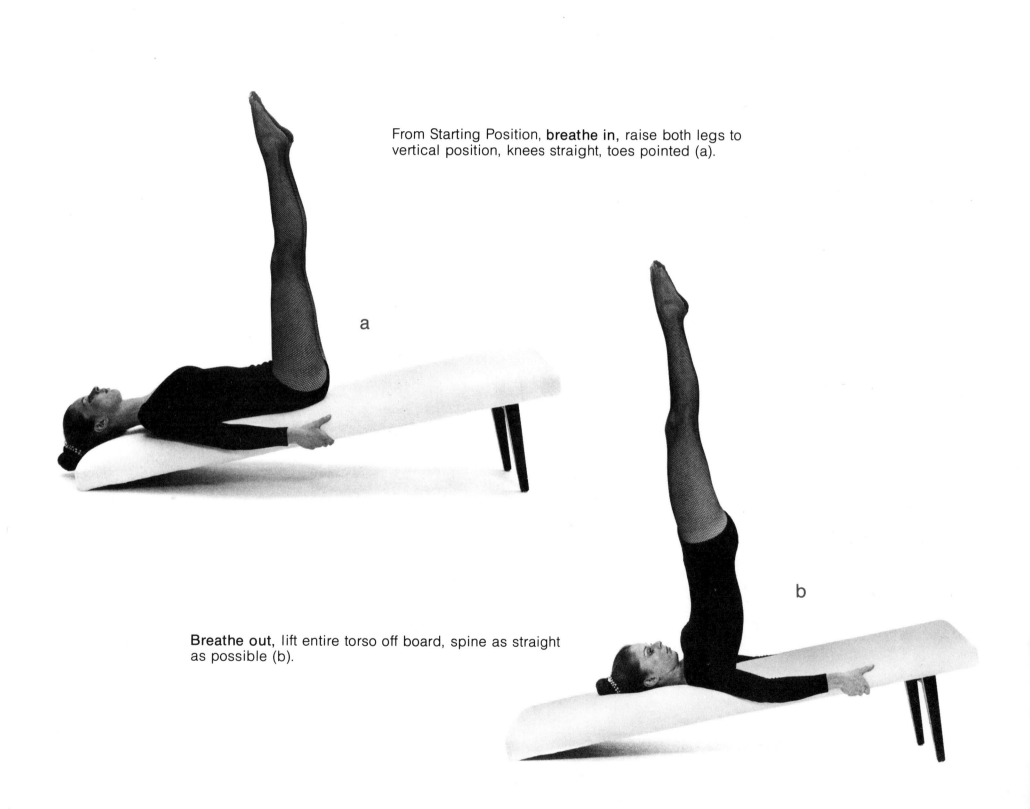

From Starting Position, **breathe in,** raise both legs to vertical position, knees straight, toes pointed (a).

a

Breathe out, lift entire torso off board, spine as straight as possible (b).

b

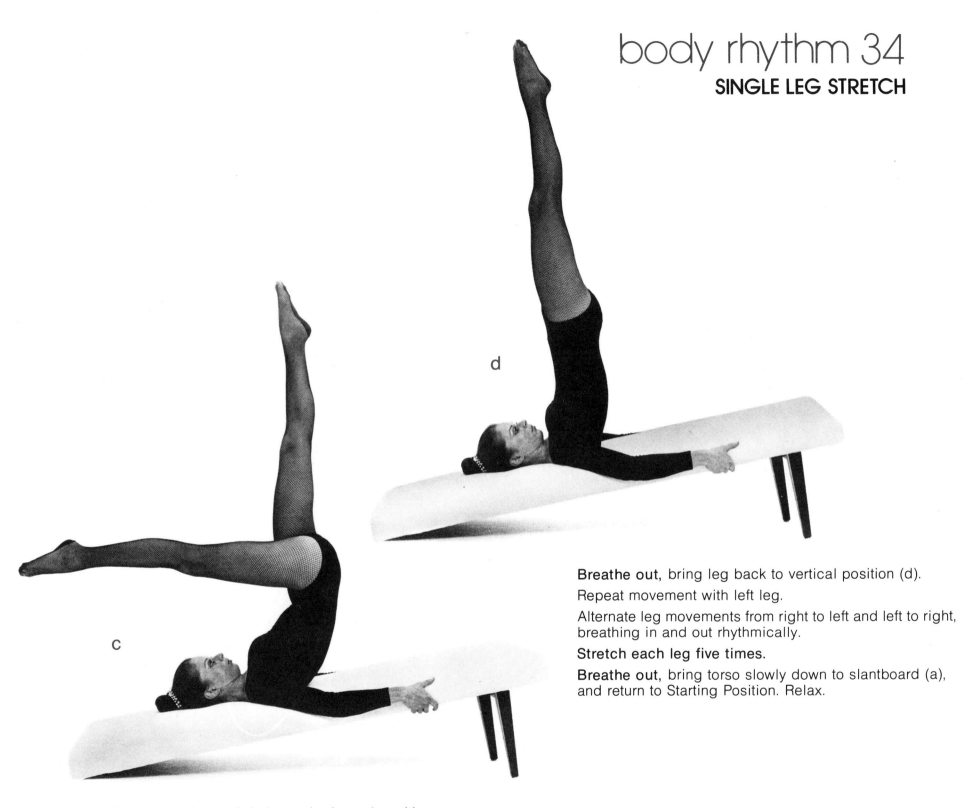

d

c

Breathe out, bring leg back to vertical position (d).

Repeat movement with left leg.

Alternate leg movements from right to left and left to right, breathing in and out rhythmically.

Stretch each leg five times.

Breathe out, bring torso slowly down to slantboard (a), and return to Starting Position. Relax.

Breathe in, lower right leg to horizontal position over head (c).

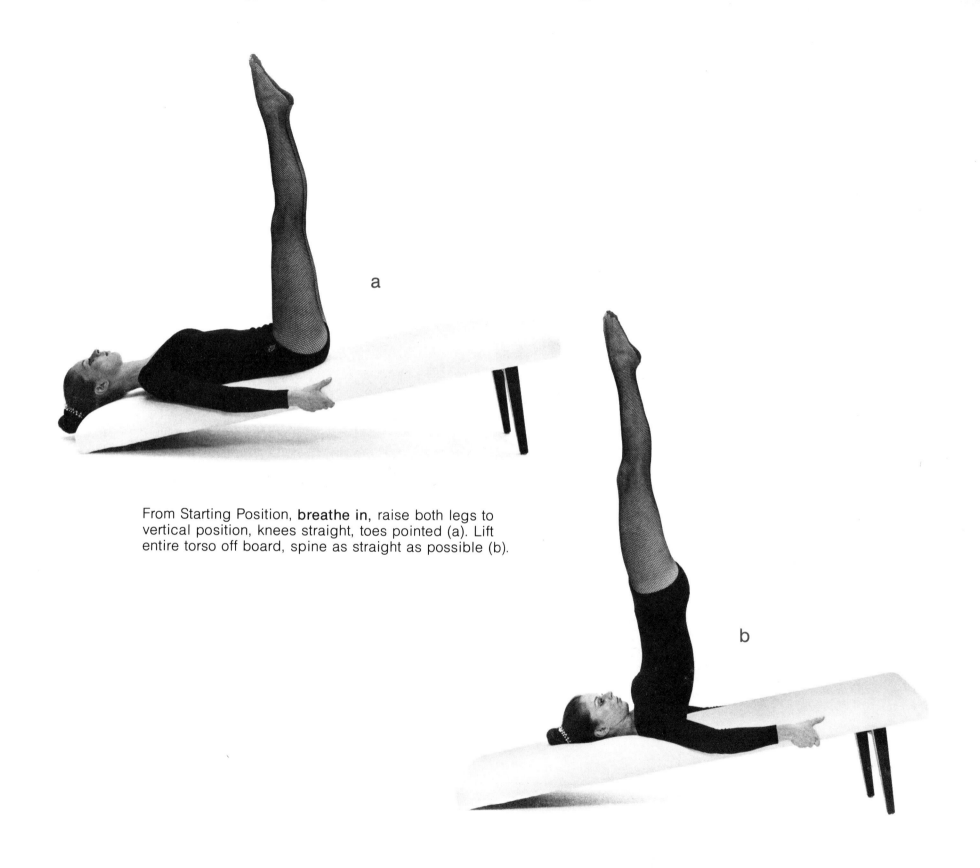

From Starting Position, **breathe in,** raise both legs to vertical position, knees straight, toes pointed (a). Lift entire torso off board, spine as straight as possible (b).

DOUBLE LEG STRETCH

Moving from hip joints, lower both legs to horizontal position over head (c).

Stretch both legs slowly over head with toes aiming down as far as possible (d).

Breathe out and slowly return legs to vertical position (b).

Breathe in, bring torso slowly down to slantboard (a), and return to Starting Position. Relax.

Repeat five times.

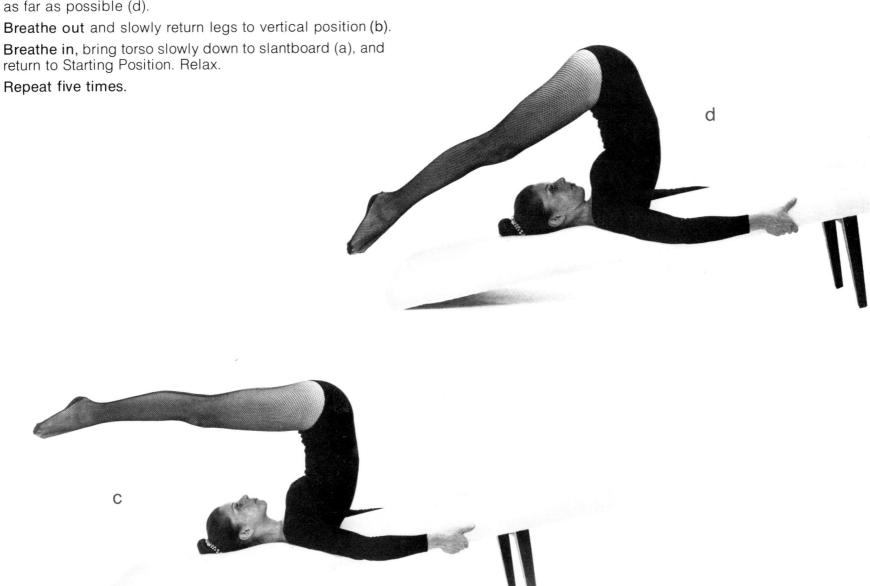

d

c

95

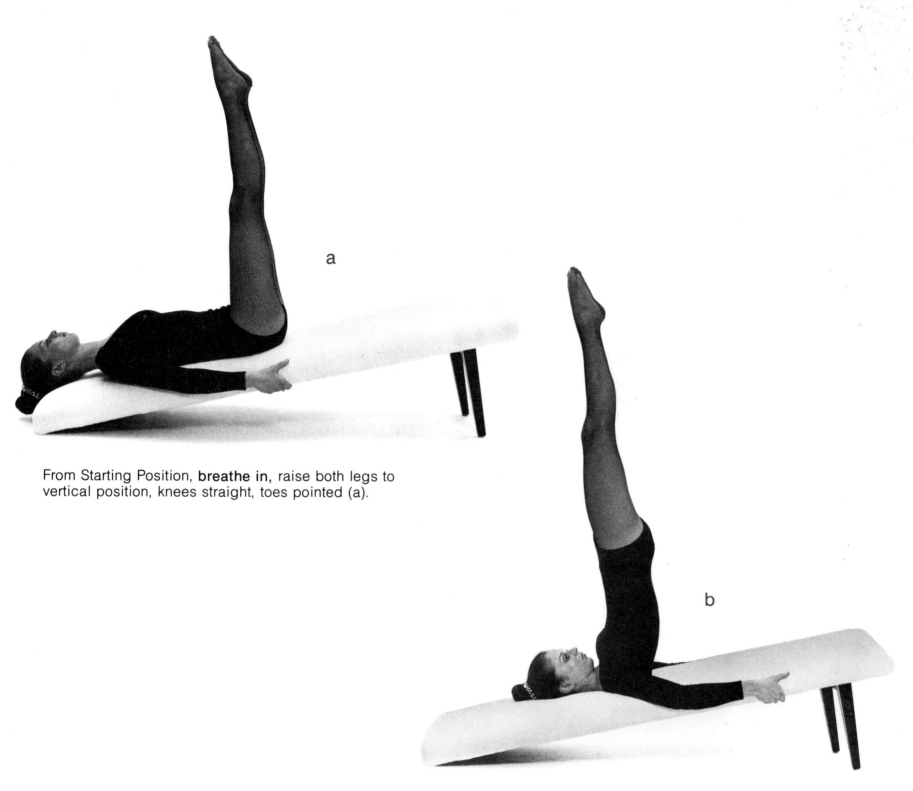

From Starting Position, **breathe in,** raise both legs to
vertical position, knees straight, toes pointed (a).

Breathe out, lift entire torso off board, spine as straight
as possible (b).

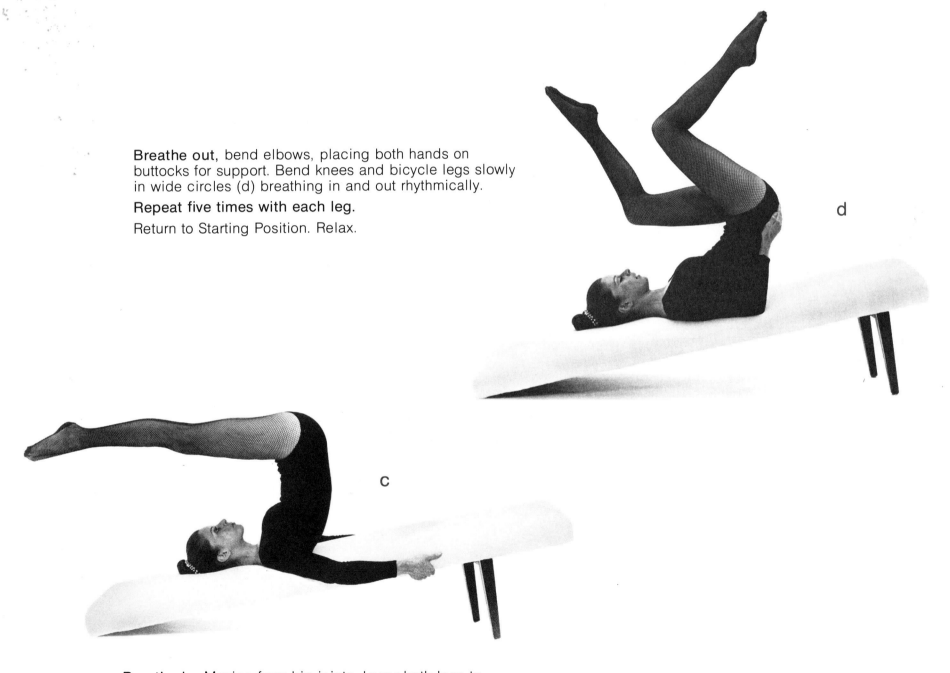

Breathe out, bend elbows, placing both hands on buttocks for support. Bend knees and bicycle legs slowly in wide circles (d) breathing in and out rhythmically.

Repeat five times with each leg.

Return to Starting Position. Relax.

d

c

Breathe in. Moving from hip joints, lower both legs to horizontal position over head (c).

body rhythms to limber spinal

column and to firm abdomen

(37-43)

These intermediate movements are designed to create elasticity in the lower back by thoroughly stretching the lumbar region of the spine and strengthening the abdominal muscles simultaneously.

Performed on a flat surface, the movements will take time to accomplish. You may find them more difficult than the previous group performed on the slantboard.

body rhythm 37

PENDULUM I

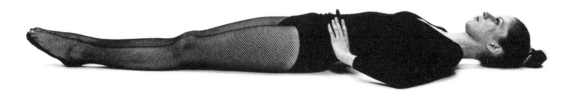

STARTING POSITION

Lie flat on floor on a mat two or three inches thick. Press lower back into mat, keeping knees straight, toes pointed. Place hands on waistline.

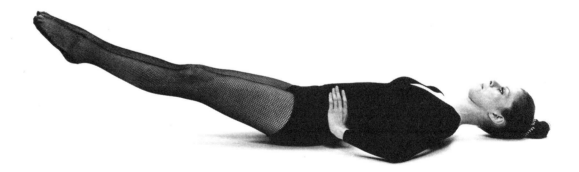

From Starting Position, **breathe in** and lift both legs about 15 inches from mat. Hold position for three seconds.

Breathe out. Return to Starting Position. Relax.

Repeat five times.

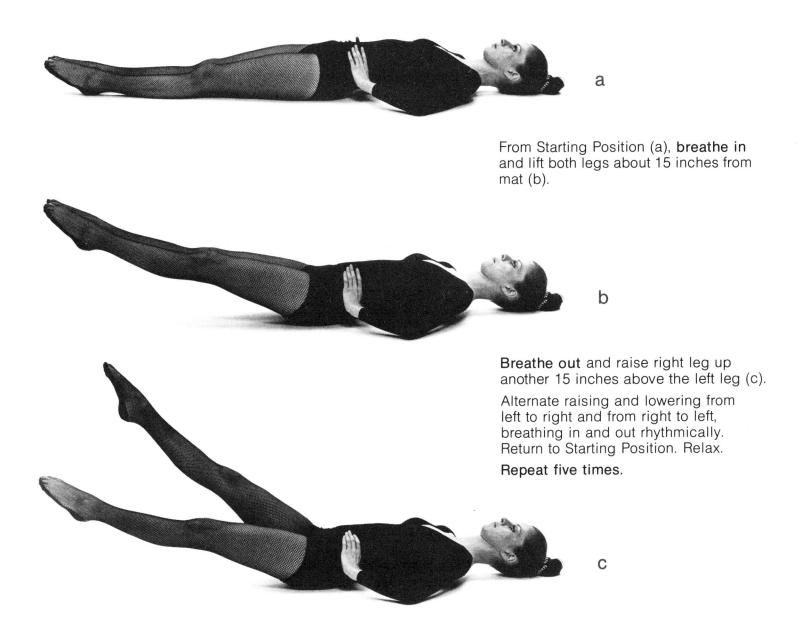

a

From Starting Position (a), **breathe in** and lift both legs about 15 inches from mat (b).

b

Breathe out and raise right leg up another 15 inches above the left leg (c).

Alternate raising and lowering from left to right and from right to left, breathing in and out rhythmically. Return to Starting Position. Relax.

Repeat five times.

c

a

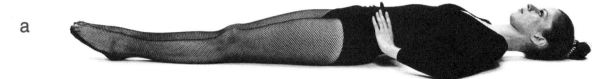

From Starting Position (a), place both palms in back of head.

b

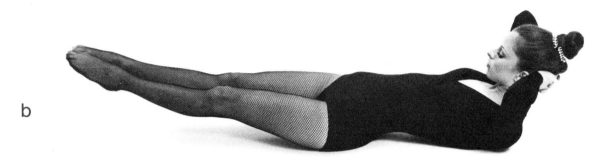

Breathe in and lift head up stretching from neckline, keeping shoulders on the mat while simultaneously lifting both legs about 15 inches off the mat (b).

c

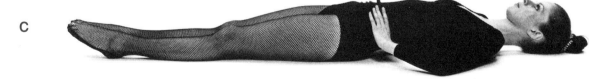

Breathe out. Return to Starting Position (c). Relax.

Repeat five times.

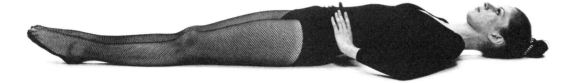

a

From Starting Position (a), place palms in back of head.

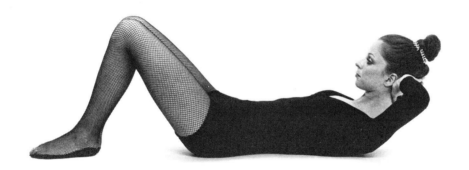

b

Bend knees and place feet flat on mat. **Breathe in** and lift head stretching from neckline keeping shoulders on the mat (b).

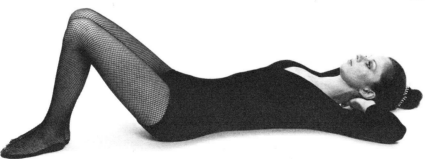

c

Breathe out while bringing head down (c). Relax.

Repeat five times.

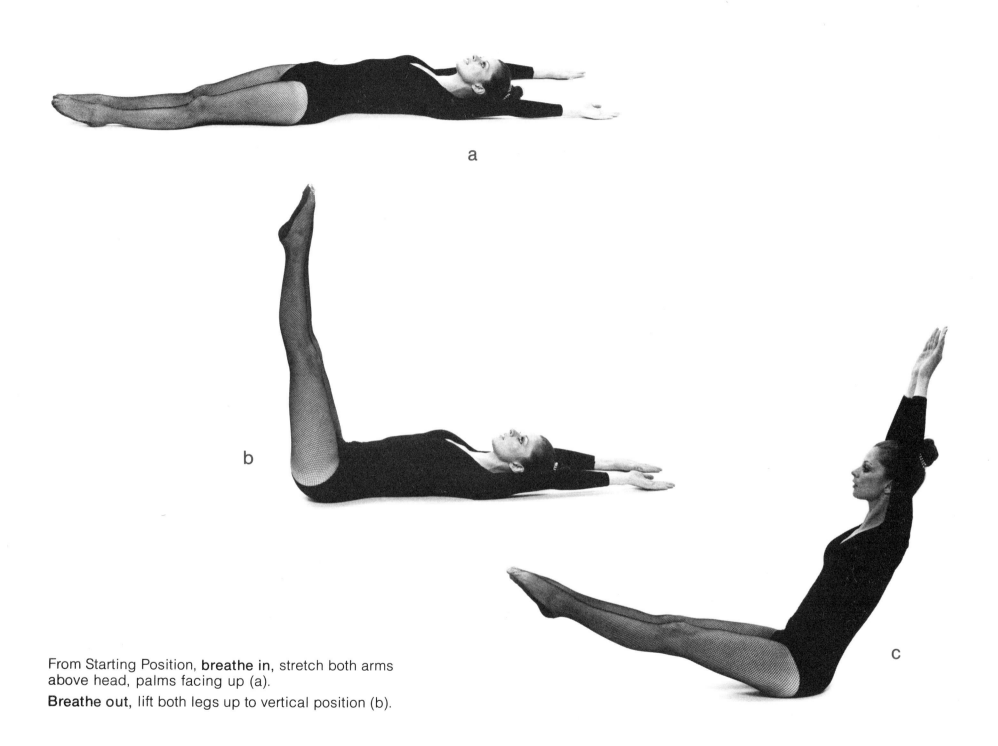

a

b

c

From Starting Position, **breathe in,** stretch both arms above head, palms facing up (a).

Breathe out, lift both legs up to vertical position (b).

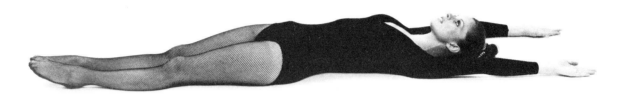

e

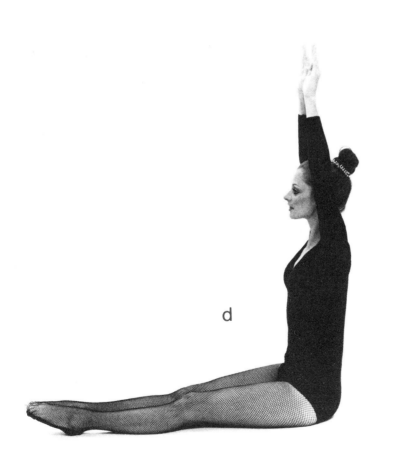

d

Breathe in, lift entire torso, moving from hip joints, off mat while lowering both legs simultaneously until you reach a sitting position with hands stretched above head (c, d).

Breathe out. Slowly return to Starting Position by lowering your torso back to mat (e). Relax.

Repeat five times.

103

a

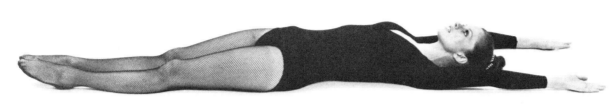

From Starting Position, stretch both arms above head, palms facing up (a).

Breathe in and stretch torso up to a sitting position (b).

Breathe out and lower both arms to shoulder level (c).

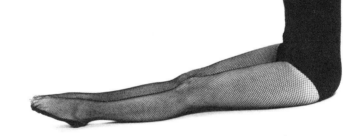

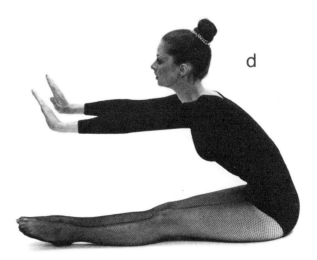

b

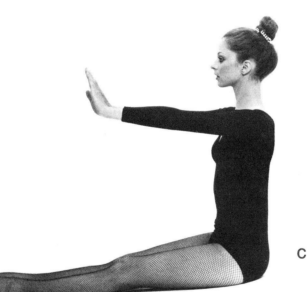

c

d

Breathe in and stretch entire torso forward moving from hip joints, knees straight, toes pointed (d). Bounce torso back and forth from hip joints three times. **Breathe out**. Return to (c). Relax.

Repeat torso bends five times from sitting position.

body rhythm 43

PENDULUM VII

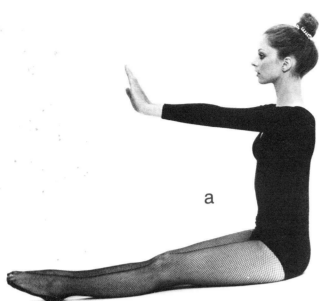

a

From a sitting position (a), stretch both legs apart, knees straight, toes pointed.

Breathe in and stretch torso forward moving from hip joints (b). Bounce torso back and forth from hip joints three times.

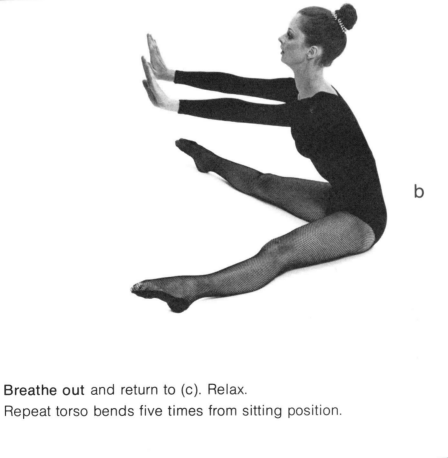

b

Breathe out and return to (c). Relax.

Repeat torso bends five times from sitting position.

c

advanced body rhythms

body rhythms for grace,

coordination

and rhythm (44-55)

The following 12 movements, performed in a kneeling position, will activate every muscle in the body.

These Body Rhythms will create flexibility in the joints and will strengthen legs and feet to make walking a pleasurable experience.

After you have mastered the advanced routines, you may enjoy practicing Body Rhythms to music. Choose a slow waltz with an even beat to help coordinate the movements.

Body Rhythm 44 is a preliminary movement designed to limber the hip joints to prepare you for these advanced routines. It is also important for proper walking, which is achieved by swinging the thighs and legs from hip joints rather than knee joints.

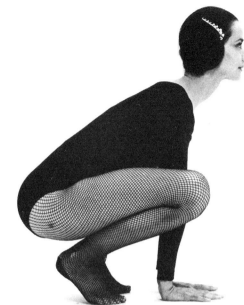

STARTING POSITION

Bend knees and lower your body to a squatting position with feet slightly apart, heels raised, arms between knees, palms flat on floor.

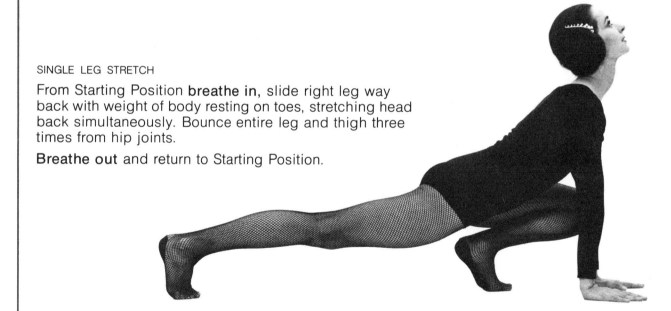

SINGLE LEG STRETCH

From Starting Position **breathe in,** slide right leg way back with weight of body resting on toes, stretching head back simultaneously. Bounce entire leg and thigh three times from hip joints.

Breathe out and return to Starting Position.

Repeat same movement with left leg.

Alternate from right to left and from left to right breathing in and out rhythmically. Return to Starting Position. Relax.

Repeat five times.

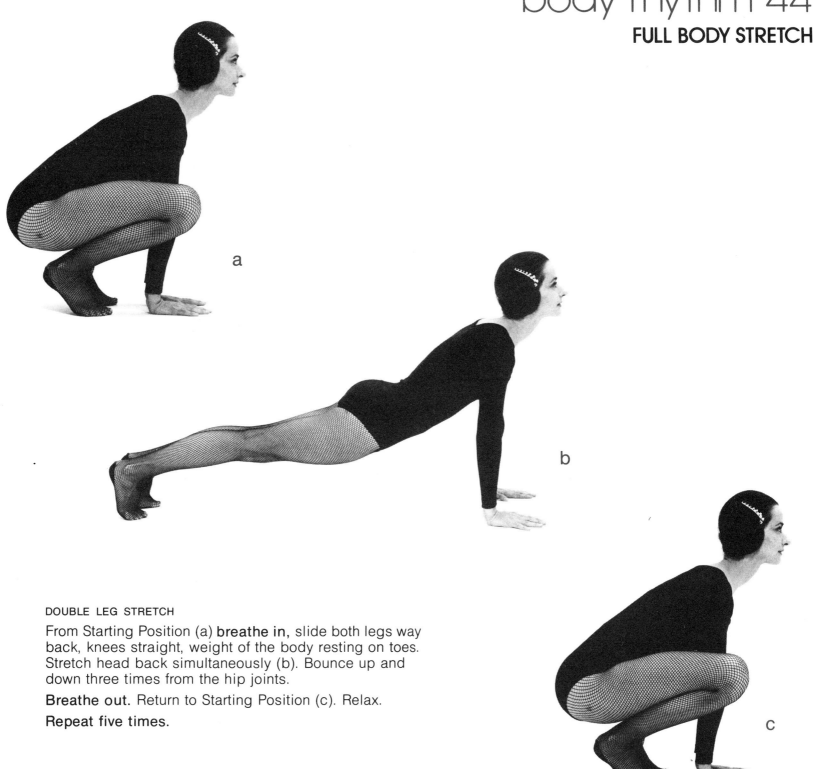

a

b

c

DOUBLE LEG STRETCH

From Starting Position (a) **breathe in,** slide both legs way back, knees straight, weight of the body resting on toes. Stretch head back simultaneously (b). Bounce up and down three times from the hip joints.

Breathe out. Return to Starting Position (c). Relax.

Repeat five times.

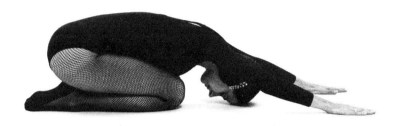

From Starting Position, **breathe in,** stretch torso upward, moving from knee joints. Bring arms to shoulder level with palms down (a).

STARTING POSITION

Kneel on mat with buttocks resting on heels. Stretch entire torso forward and down, back straight with arms stretched forward, palms touching mat.

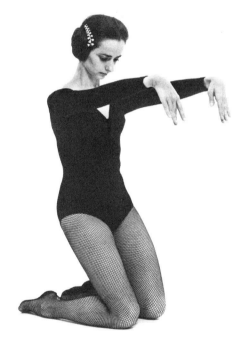

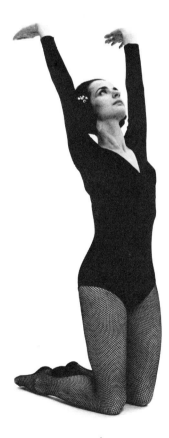

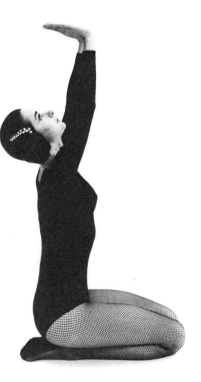

Continue to stretch torso to upright position with arms stretched above head, hands flexed with palms facing up (b).

Breathe out, moving from knee joints, return to sitting position (c). Moving from hip joints, return to Starting Position. Relax.

Repeat five times.

a

b

c

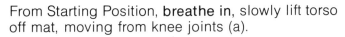

From Starting Position, **breathe in**, slowly lift torso off mat, moving from knee joints (a).

Continue to stretch body to upright position with arms slowly gliding from thighs to waistline (b), from waistline to shoulders (c).

a

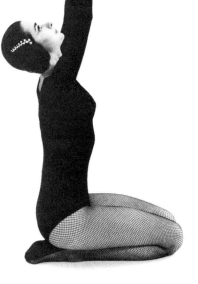

b

c

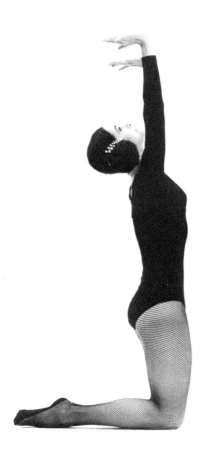

d

e

Breathe out. Stretch both arms way up, flexing hands, palms up. Bring head back simultaneously (d).

Breathe in, lower torso down with buttocks resting on heels (e).

Breathe out and lower entire body to Starting Position. Relax.

Repeat five times.

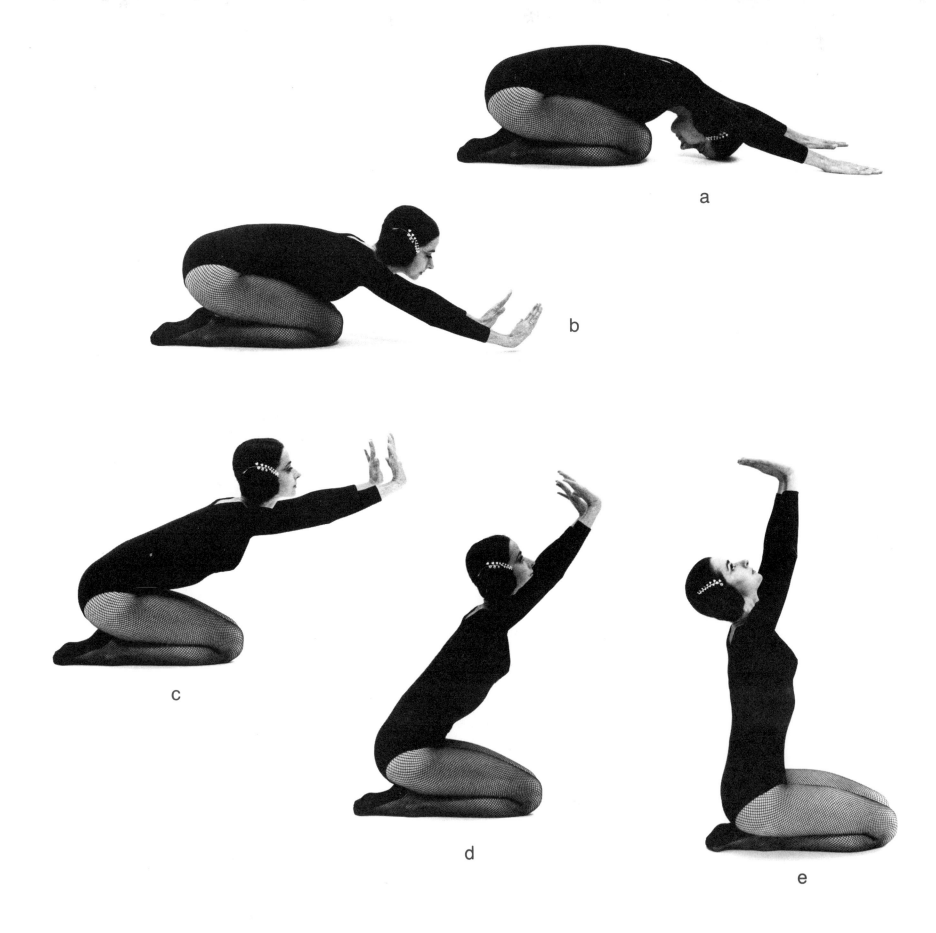

a

b

c

d

e

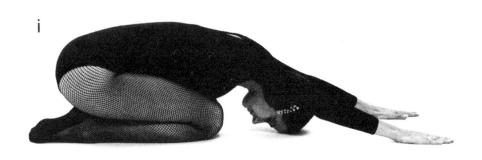

i

From Starting Position (a), **breathe in.** Lift torso, moving from hip joints, and slowly come to a sitting position with hands flexed and arms stretched above head, palms up (b, c, d, e).

Breathe out and slowly lower torso down, moving from hip joints, continuing to keep arms stretched out with palms up. Keep moving downward until you get back to Starting Position (f, g, h, i). Relax.

Repeat five times.

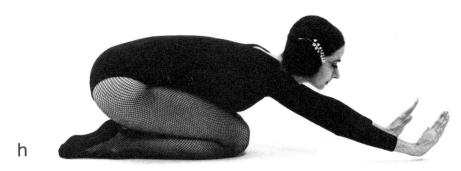

h

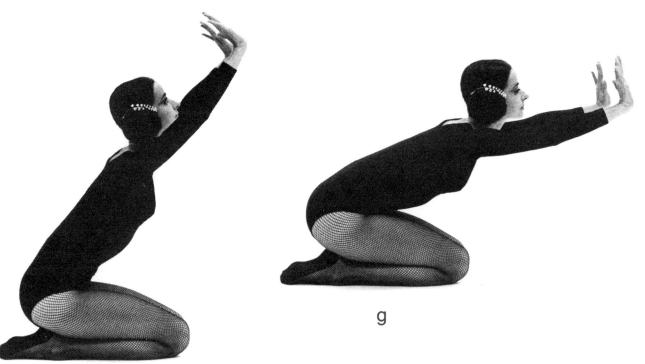

f

g

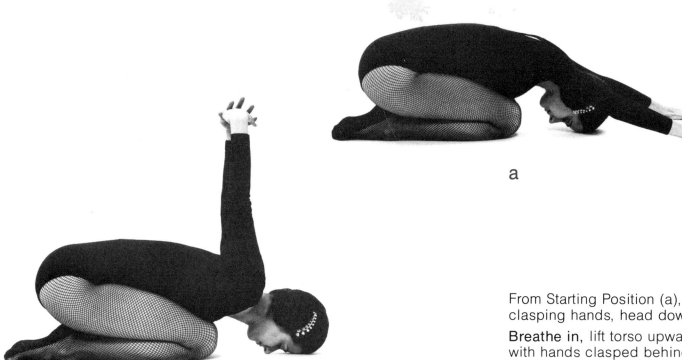

a

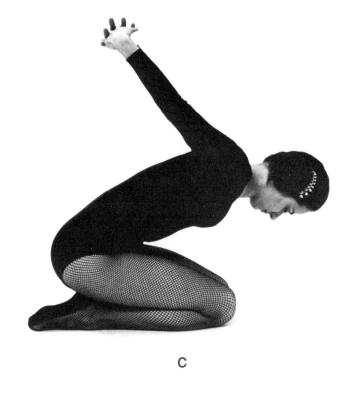

b

From Starting Position (a), stretch arms behind you, clasping hands, head down (b).

Breathe in, lift torso upward keeping head down with hands clasped behind you. Continue to stretch to upright position (c).

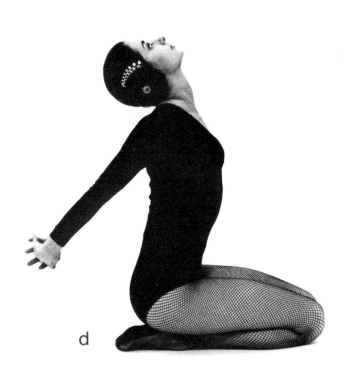

c

d

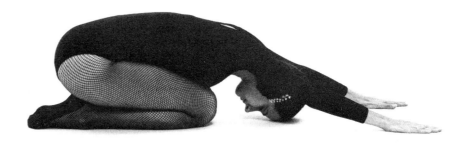

Breathe out, stretch head and arms as far back as possible (d). Return to Starting Position (e, f, g). Relax.

Repeat five times.

g

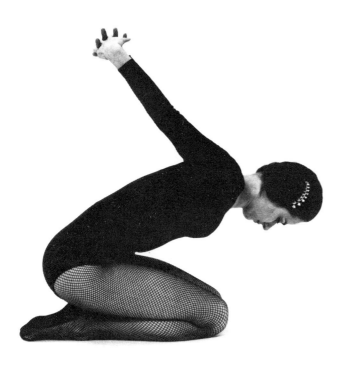

e

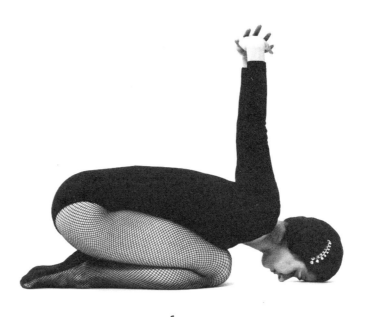

f

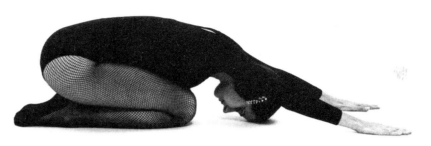

a

From Starting Position (a), stretch right leg backward, toes pointed, knee as straight as possible (b).

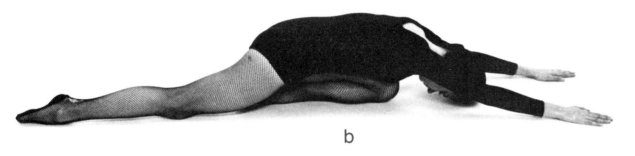

b

Breathe in, lift torso upward, slowly moving from hip joints, while keeping palms down (c).

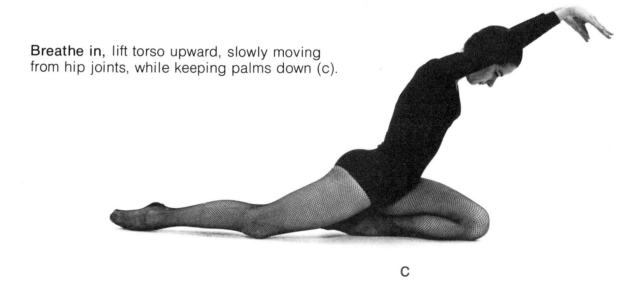

c

Breathe out, slowly bring torso back to mat (e). Return right leg to Starting Position. Relax.

Repeat entire movement with left leg. Relax.

Alternate leg movements from right to left, breathing in and out rhythmically.

Repeat five times.

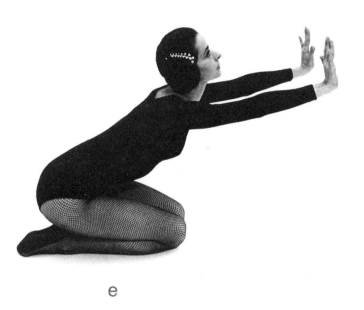

e

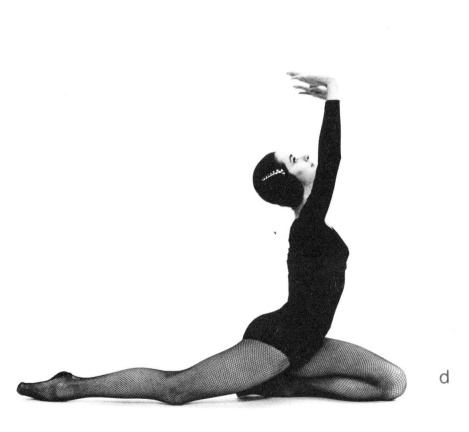

d

Stretch torso to an upright position, bring head back, and turn palms up (d).

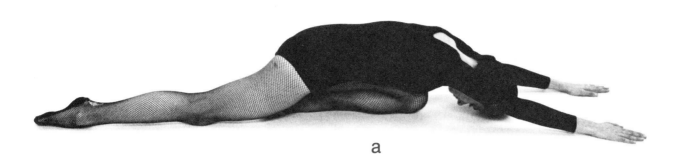

a

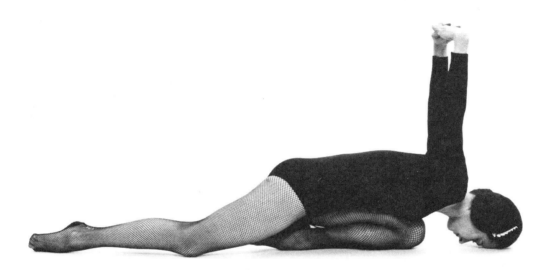

b

From Starting Position, stretch right leg
backward, toes pointed, knee straight (a).
Stretch arms behind you, clasping hands (b).

Breathe in, lift torso slowly upward to an
upright position (c, d).

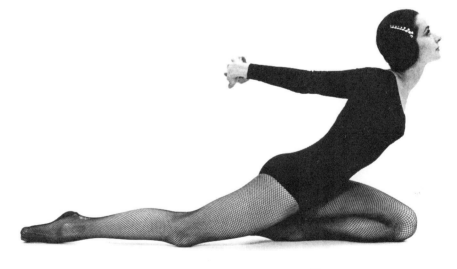

c

116

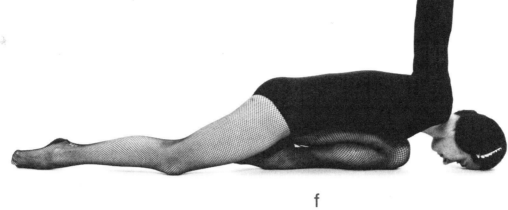

f

Breathe out and stretch both arms with clasped hands way back. Bring head back simultaneously (e, f).

Breathe in and slowly bring torso back to upright position.

Breathe out, bring torso back to mat. Return right leg to starting position. Relax.

Repeat entire movement with left leg. Relax.

Alternate leg movements from right to left, breathing in and out rhythmically.

Repeat five times.

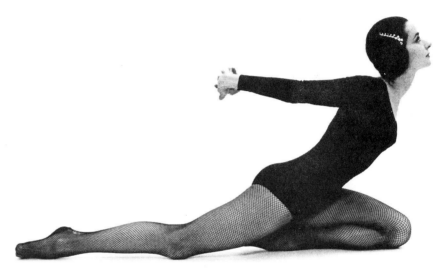

e

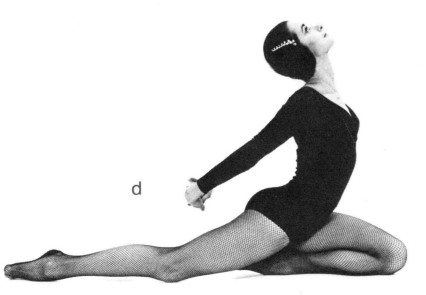

d

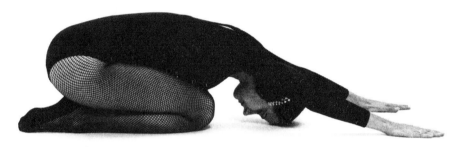

a

From Starting Position (a) **breathe in,** lift torso
moving from knee joints to a horizontal position
with palms placed on mat, elbows straight, head
stretched back (b).

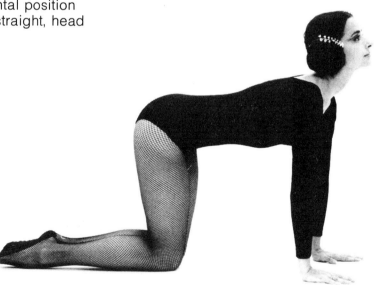

b

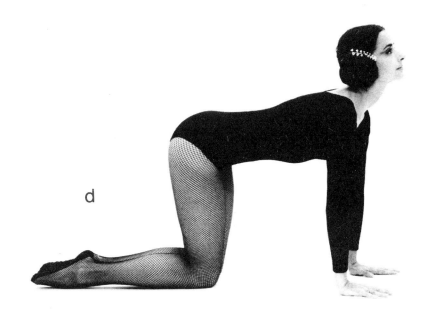

Breathe in, lift torso back to horizontal position (d).

Breathe out, lower torso to mat moving from hip joints, back straight, elbows bent, palms on mat, head facing toward left.

Breathe in, lift torso back to horizontal position (d).

Breathe out. Return to Starting Position (a). Relax.

Repeat five times.

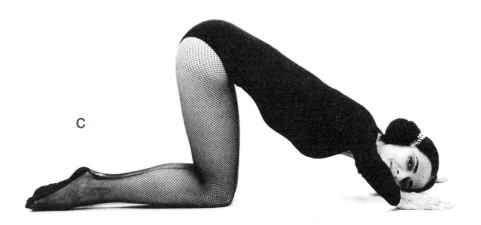

Breathe out, lower torso to mat moving from hip joints, back straight, elbows bent, palms on mat with head facing toward right (c).

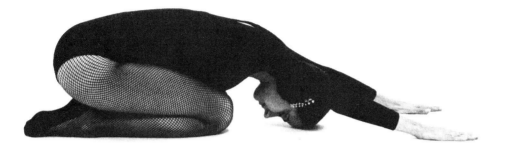

a

From Starting Position (a), **breathe in,** lift torso off mat moving from knee joints to a horizontal position with palms placed on mat, elbows straight, head stretched back (b).

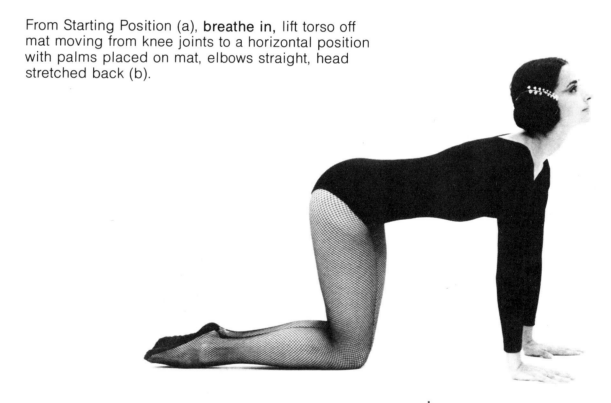

b

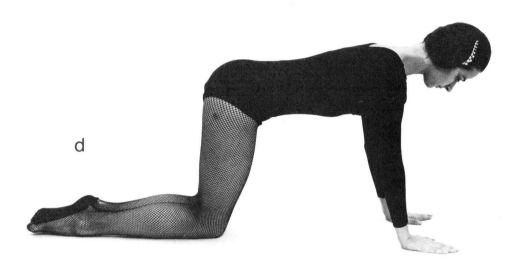

Breathe in, bend right knee and bring it back to left knee (d). Relax.

Repeat movement with left leg.

Alternate from right to left five times.

Return to Starting Position (a).

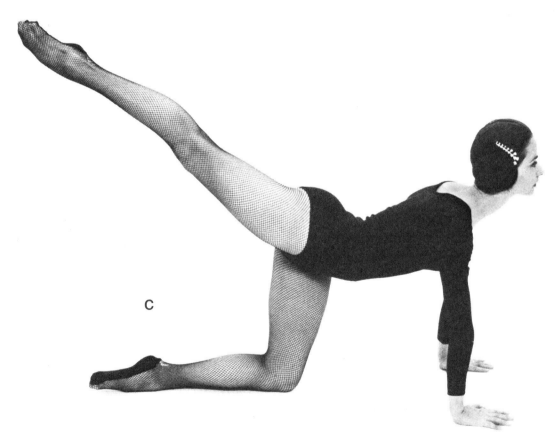

Breathe out, stretch right leg way up moving from hip joint, knee straight, toes pointed (c).

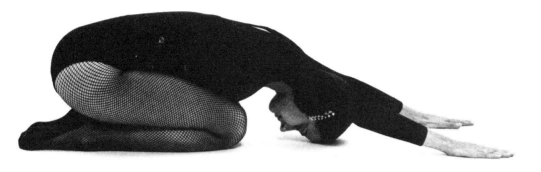

a

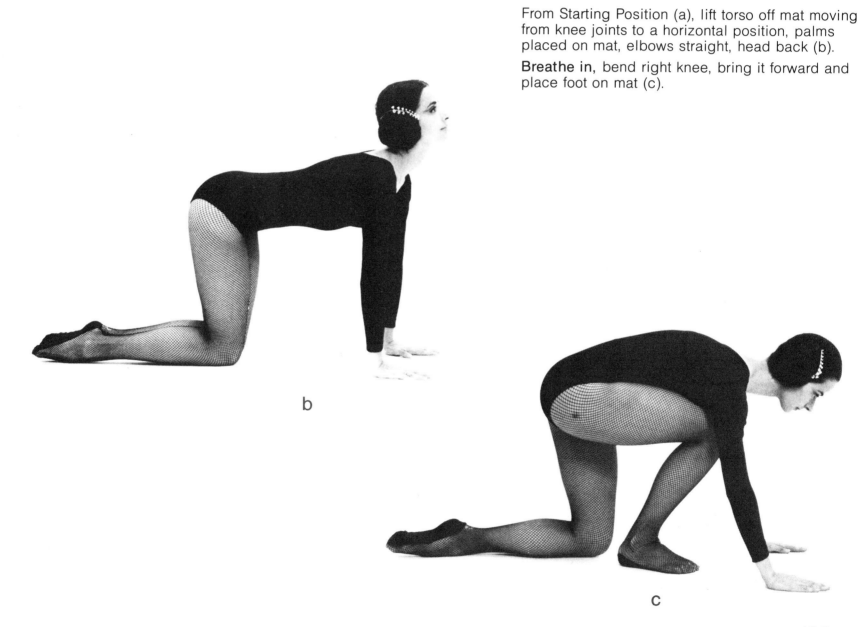

From Starting Position (a), lift torso off mat moving from knee joints to a horizontal position, palms placed on mat, elbows straight, head back (b).

Breathe in, bend right knee, bring it forward and place foot on mat (c).

b

c

122

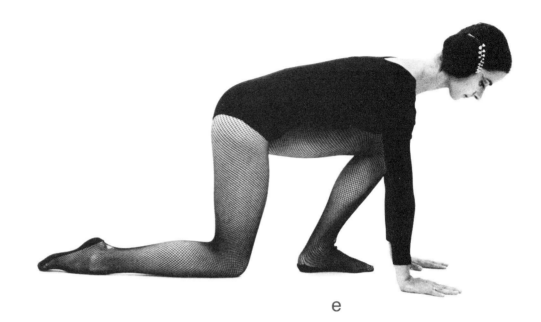

e

Breathe out and bring knee back to mat (d).

Breathe in, bend left knee, bring it forward and place left foot on mat (e).

Breathe out and bring left knee back to right knee.

Alternate movement from right to left. Relax.

Repeat five times.

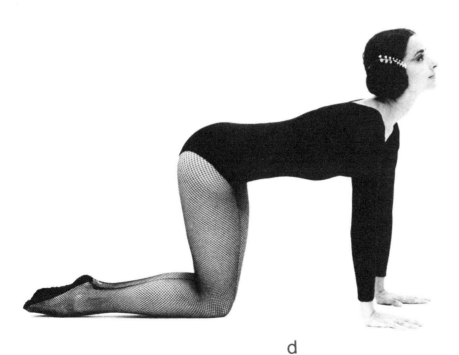

d

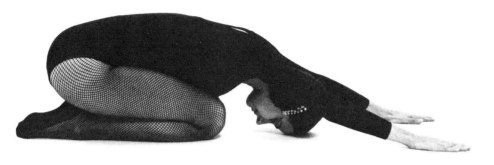

a

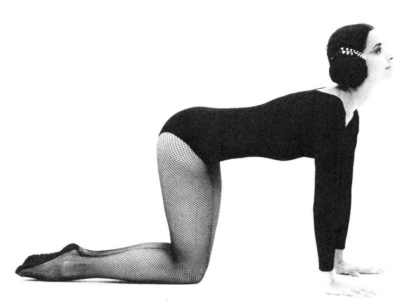

b

From Starting Position (a), **breathe in,** lift torso off mat moving from knee joints to a horizontal position with palms placed on mat, elbows straight, head back (b).

From horizontal position, **breathe out,** bend right knee, bring it forward and place foot on mat (c).

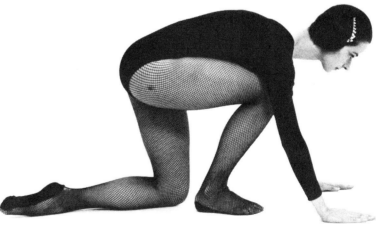

c

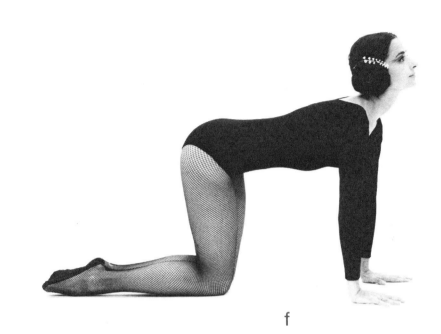

f

Breathe in, bend left knee, bring it forward and place foot on mat. Straighten out both knees as you lift torso upward keeping palms on mat, back straight (d). **Breathe out.**

Return to horizontal position by bending left knee first, right knee next (e).

Repeat same movement from horizontal position (f) five times, breathing in and out rhythmically. Relax.

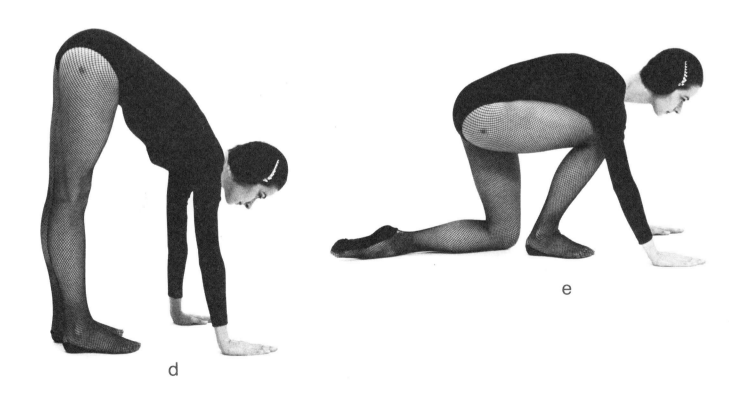

e

d

125

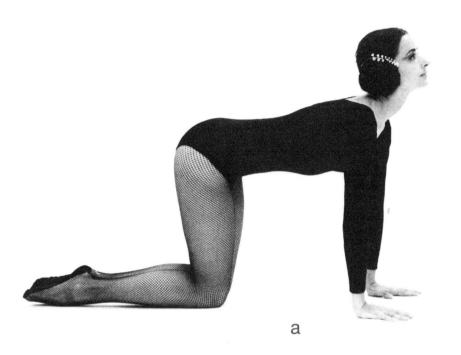

a

From horizontal position on knees (a), **breathe in,** bend right knee, bring it forward, and place foot on mat (b).

Breathe out, bend left knee, bring it forward, place foot on mat. Straighten both knees as you lift torso up, keeping palms on mat, back straight (c).

Breathe in, raise torso to horizontal position, moving from hip joints (d).

Breathe out, lower torso, moving from hip joints, placing palms on mat (c). Relax.

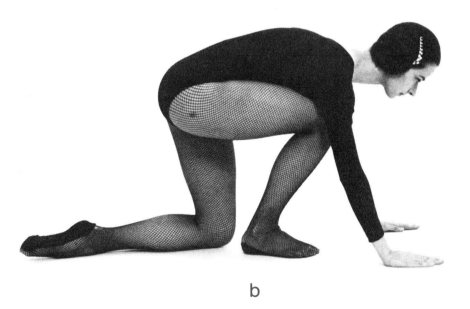

b

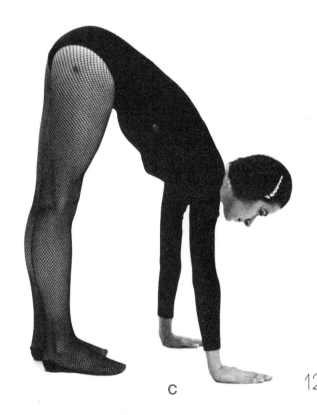

c

126

Repeat five times by returning to horizontal position (d).

From horizontal position (d), **breathe in,** stretch torso up, moving from hip joints, with elbows straight, arms high above head with palms turned toward ceiling (e).

Breathe out and return to horizontal position (d). Relax.

Repeat five times.

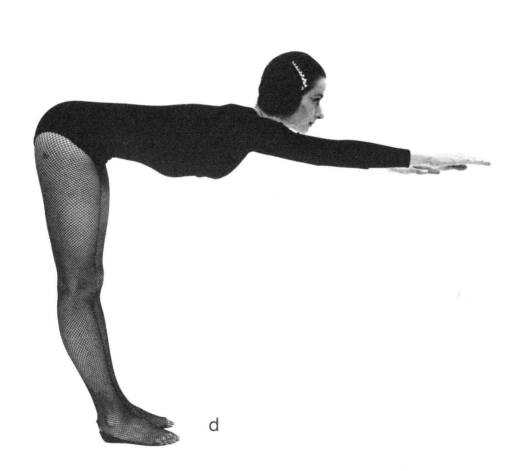

d

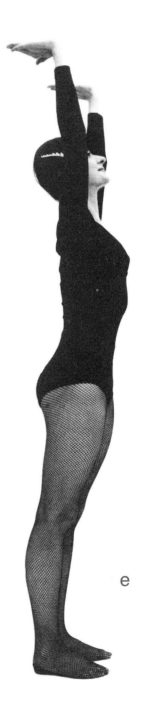

e

nutrition and diet

knowing how to eat makes all the difference

Not too many years ago, three "square" meals a day was considered standard eating practice. Today the standard is more like a skipped breakfast, lunch on the run, a starch-heavy dinner and snacks, snacks, snacks in between. What a sorry state of eating we're in! Despite the wealth of the country and the tremendous advances we have made in the field of nutrition, we are a nation of poor eaters. Even the affluent suffer from malnutrition. American eating habits are so bad, in fact, that faulty nutrition is one of our most pressing national health problems.

Did you know, for example, that 30 percent of Americans are overweight, and an even greater number are underweight? The frightening number of illnesses associated with poor nutrition include heart disease; diabetes; dysfunctions of the liver, kidney, and gall bladder; anemia; tooth decay; hypoglycemia; and even mental and behavioral aberrations.

To what do we owe this unhappy state of affairs? The answer is simple—a lack of knowledge about all-important nutrition. Our medical community has not yet made the transition from curative medicine to preventive medicine. And proper nutrition is preventive medicine, indeed!

The average person knows very little about what should and, indeed, *must* be eaten if he is to remain healthy and energetic. Most people indulge far too much in "junk food"—snack items and prepared foods that are full of preservatives, additives, sugar, and fat. One shocking recent statistic tells us that sugar consumption has risen to an extraordinary 120 pounds per person each year!

A sad and ironic result of our nutrition ignorance is that great numbers of obese teenagers in the United States are actually suffering from malnutrition. For this to happen in a country of such abundance is indeed a tragedy. Plump but undernourished children result from parents who have overlooked the importance of certain food groups and have allowed their children to load up on junk foods. Why? Because we have severely neglected our education in the field of nutrition. If you are one of the people who eats great quantities of food, yet starves your body of the essential elements that build good health, you must take the time to learn that less can be more. By making careful choices, you can thrive on smaller but more nourishing quantities and improve not only your general health, but your appearance as well.

The basis of a healthy diet is eating proper amounts from each of five main food groups. This is important because each group has a distinct function necessary to your complete nourishment. Try to understand this principle. It will help you plan a sound, healthful diet to meet your daily needs.

avoid fad diets

Most fad diets call for the elimination of one or more of the basic food groups. Not only is this unwise, it is downright dangerous! Your body needs nourishment from each and every group, no matter what you weigh. Even while purporting to help you, fad diets, which are usually crash diets, run completely against nature's basic requirements for sustaining good health and stamina. Because they fail to provide adequate nourishment, they often cause malnutrition. Aside from being unnatural, fad diets are generally of short duration and, at best, give only temporary results. And if followed for prolonged periods, they can not only lessen vitality and break down resistance to disease, they can even ruin a perfectly good disposition! No matter how you look at it, fad diets are a sure way to hasten old age.

As in so many phases in life, it is quality, not quantity, in food that counts. You have got to come to terms with the fact that you will never get any permanent results from dieting unless you choose a program that can remain the basis of changed eating habits for the rest of your life. Only a food program that is varied, regulated, selected from balanced food groups, and faithfully followed can give you long-range satisfaction and lasting results.

the facts about nutrition

Understanding the following facts about nutrition will help you make more intelligent use of the meals and diets coming up later in this section. There are five basic food groups: proteins, carbohydrates, fats, vitamins, and minerals. I am going to explain these groups, make clear why they are so necessary, and point out which foods are highly nourishing. You will be pleasantly surprised at the great number of tasty foods you will find, foods you actually like but may have left out of your diet or eaten only occasionally, due to carelessness or lack of knowledge.

Proteins Proteins build and revitalize tissues to keep your body in good overall condition. They are the main substance found in muscles, organs, skin, hair, and other tissues. Your blood must have proteins, and even your bones, teeth, and nails need some. Proteins also help form many vital glandular secretions and certain infection-fighting substances. Found in both animal and plant foods, the better-quality protein comes from the following two groups:

GROUP A includes meat, fish, and dairy products, such as liver, cheese, whole milk, skim milk, buttermilk, and yogurt.

GROUP B includes, among other things, soybeans, whole grain cereals (especially oatmeal), coarse breads, dried peas and beans, lima beans, peanuts and other nuts, and peanut butter.

Because protein is never stored in the body, you must eat some every day. Of the five essential food groups, protein is the one needed most and in the largest quantities. Proteins actually help consume the carbohydrates, fats, and acids in the body, and adult women, no matter what their level of activity, should eat no less than 240 calories (60 grams) of protein a day.

Carbohydrates Carbohydrates, what we commonly think of as starches and sweets, provide the body with energy to work, to play, and even to sleep soundly. They are found in a great variety of foods, including bread, crackers, cereals, macaroni, spaghetti, noodles, potatoes, rice, flour; starchy vegetables like peas, beans, etc.; dried fruits; sugars and sweets, such as honey, molasses, jams, jellies, and syrups. These foods produce heat and energy, but turn into fats and acids in the body if consumed in great quantities. We generally get ample carbohydrates without even trying, since most basic foods contain carbohydrates in satisfactory amounts. When we indulge in too many carbohydrates, however, the surplus is stored in the body as fat. That is why so many reducers cut them out entirely, which is a mistake. If you do this, proteins will be diverted from their main function in the body—upkeep and repair—and be forced to supply the needed energy. This is a well-known fact. The sensible thing to do is to *control* your intake of carbohydrates instead of *eliminating them altogether.*

Fats Like carbohydrates, fats provide energy, and what is not used up through activity or thrown off is stored in the body as fat. Found in butter and margarine, egg yolks, cream, salad and cooking oils, cheese made from whole milk or cream, bacon and other fat meat, mayonnaise, and nuts, fats are another food group mistakenly avoided by reducers. Again, intake should be controlled and not cut out entirely.

Minerals Although they are needed only in small quantities, minerals play a vital part in helping the body to work normally. An adequately balanced diet of high protein foods should provide enough of all minerals. Deficiencies of calcium, iron, and iodine are relatively common, however, and should be watched for.

CALCIUM The mineral that promotes strong bones and teeth, helps muscles to contract and relax, keeps nerves in good shape, and regulates the heartbeat is found in both milk and green-leafed vegetables.

PHOSPHORUS This mineral helps maintain bones and teeth by assisting in the proper utilization of calcium; it also helps carbohydrates produce energy and keeps the blood alkaline. It is found in milk, eggs, fish, lean meats, poultry, soybeans, cereals, and breads.

IRON This is one of the materials essential to the red blood cells. It provides color for complexion and general vitality. It is found in lean meats in general, especially liver, heart, and kidneys, as well as in a variety of other foods like green-leafed vegetables, egg yolks, whole grain bread and cereals, molasses, dried apricots, peaches, and oysters.

IODINE Besides increasing the body's alertness and efficiency, iodine helps the functioning of the thyroid gland, which controls many of the body's chemical processes. It is found in seafood and in iodized salt.

Vitamins Actually chemical compounds found in minute quantities in foods, vitamins protect your overall health and ward off certain diseases. While building the strength of the nervous system, they also help to derive the utmost in nourishment from foods. *Caution:* Supplements in the form of vitamin concentrates should be used only on the advice of a doctor.

VITAMIN A This important vitamin keeps your skin, eyes, glands, and mucous membranes healthy; helps you resist colds and other respiratory infections; and helps the body utilize calcium and iron. Vitamin A is found in dark green leafy vegetables, yellow vegetables and fruits, liver, egg yolk, yellow cheese, butter and fortified margarine, cream and whole milk.

VITAMIN B_1 Besides stimulating the appetite, B_1 keeps the digestive and nervous systems in good order, keeps the mind alert, prevents fatigue and irritability, and helps the body utilize carbohydrates, hence adding energy. It is found in meats such as liver, heart, kidneys, ham, lamb, veal, lean beef, and poultry, and in fish, eggs, green peas, beans, whole grain and enriched grain products, peanuts and other nuts, and milk.

VITAMIN B_2 (RIBOFLAVIN) In making you more vigorous by helping the body to utilize carbohydrates and fats, B_2 influences the nervous system, digestion, and general body resistance to disease. It is found in all vegetables, green beans and peas, whole grain and enriched bread, and cereals (especially oatmeal), soybean products, and dried beans.

NIACIN This third member of the Vitamin B family helps digestion and protects nerve tissue, thus helping mental balance. It is found in liver, lean meat, poultry, tuna fish, salmon, sardines, and other fish, peanut butter, soybean products, whole grain and enriched cereals and breads, molasses, grits, and enriched cornmeal.

VITAMIN C Also known as ascorbic acid, Vitamin C builds strong blood vessels and healthy gums, helps the body resist infection, helps cuts and wounds heal more quickly, and strengthens teeth, bones, blood vessels, and muscles. It is found in citrus fruits and tomatoes, green-leafed vegetables, vegetable juices, cantaloupe and other melons, strawberries, blackberries, raspberries, blueberries, potatoes, and raw apples.

VITAMIN D The "sunshine" vitamin helps the body utilize calcium and phosphorus, thus increasing the strength of bones and teeth. Vitamin D is found in eggs, fish roe, mackerel, fish-liver oils, and milk fortified with Vitamin D. It is also absorbed through the skin from direct sunshine.

Some vitamins are easily destroyed by heat or air; others dissolve in fat or water. Whenever possible, then, you should eat vitamin-rich foods raw. If you must cook them, do it for as short a time as possible, in as little water as needed, and in tightly covered pots.

Notice how often many of the same foods appear again and again in the lists of the five essentials to good health. Perhaps you understand now more fully why it is important in planning a diet, to include selections from each of these groups—whether you are overweight, or underweight, or even if your weight is ideal. The best diet, in any case, is one that is good for your health, as well as for regulating your weight.

Food intake, of course, must be guided by need. It stands to reason, for example, that a young child will need smaller portions of everything, except of milk, than a teenager. A nursing mother, or a very active man or woman, will require the most. Less generous servings, of course, go also to older people because they become less active, and past the age of fifty, the body's need for fuel diminishes.

what about calories?

This brings us to the subject of calories. They are, by definition, the measurement of the energy which a certain quantity of food is capable of producing. The calorie is used to express the heat output of an organism and the fuel or energy value of food. If you are large, active, or still growing, or have big bones or engage actively in sports or any regular outdoor physical labor, it stands to reason you will need more calories than if you are small and inclined toward a sedentary way of life.

Calories are like the fuel for a car or any other machine, except that, in this case, there is a danger of overfueling. To most people, calories are not only confusing, they are annoying. It is certainly unpleasant to eat your way through your meals with a calorie counter checking each item for its caloric value. The bet-

ter way is to let someone else do the counting and planning for you, and that is exactly what I've done with my specific day-to-day menus. All based on formulas for correct nutritional balance, they are worked out for individual specific weight problems whether you plan to lose, gain, or maintain your ideal weight.

the right diet for you

In the simplest terms: If you want to lose weight, your daily intake should be a little below normal. If you are overweight, no matter how serious the problem may appear, you need enough of the right foods to provide energy for your daily activities. If you are underweight and want to gain, your intake should be above normal, but consisting of foods that will build muscle tissue and not fat. Whatever your problem, the first thing you must learn to do is become portion-conscious. Even a strict diet should never make you feel unhappy, or give you that sense of deprivation that so many unnecessarily strict routines do.

This puts everything on the wrong footing, because the unpleasant feeling of having things taken away often weakens willpower and becomes the deciding influence in making you break your diet. A good diet should be considered not a "minus," but a "plus." The ideal diet should provide added strength, as well as weight loss, and pleasure instead of depression. It needn't be a skimpy, raw-celery-and-fruit affair, nor does it have to be a monotonous bore.

New habits take time   It is important to face the fact that a successful change of eating habits takes time. In some cases, it may take a week or longer on a proper diet before any change becomes noticeable. You should never expect to lose more than two pounds per week; and only a long-term, proper diet will bring long-term results.

Weigh yourself every morning, using the same scale each day. If there is no change, you can easily adjust the quantity of food you consume. Remember, proper dieting is based on proper eating patterns, and, once adopted, they can easily be maintained for a lifetime of good nutrition.

Although vitamins are essential to an adequate diet, they are

something we have grown to think of as extraneous materials that come from the drugstore. Drugstore vitamins are *supplementary,* and, while beneficial, they are not a substitute for food. Our best bets for natural vitamins are the butcher, the grocer, and the fruit and vegetable market.

On the whole, it is best to avoid as much as possible foods that are canned, preserved, pickled, bottled, bleached, polished, or refined. Other foods to say no to are white flour, white rice, white sugar, cocoa and chocolate, coffee, and alcohol, all of which are lacking in nutrients and are often even obstructive to the proper absorption and utilization of nutrients from other sources. For good health, say yes to whole grain flour, brown rice, honey, fresh fruit, fresh vegetables, and various milk products such as buttermilk, cottage cheese, yogurt, and skimmed milk.

If you are on a really strict reducing diet, choose vegetables from those with low sugar content and the fewest calories—lettuce, cucumbers, spinach, asparagus, escarole, endive, Swiss chard, celery, tomatoes, watercress, kale, cauliflower, eggplant, cabbage, radishes, leeks, string beans, and broccoli. Select low sugar fruits from among this group: grapefruit, oranges, tangerines, pineapples, melons, pears, plums, apricots, apples, peaches, currants, cranberries, strawberries, blueberries, and cherries.

Because your body works best on a schedule, it is a good idea to have a regular time each day for elimination. Refined and denatured foods, besides being non-nutritious, are acid-forming, and leave very little of the cellulose residue the colon needs to induce proper elimination. Instead, you need whole grain breads and cereals, fresh vegetables and fruits. These good foods contribute the fiber and bulk which make digestion and elimination a smooth and natural process. For the constipation problems that many Americans suffer from, pills and powders offer temporary relief. But sensible eating, coupled with special abdominal exercises (see Body Rhythms 1–6), is a more realistic antidote.

Some people find it easier to diet in summer when the weather and available foods are more conducive to eating less heavily. Others claim that midwinter, particularly after the holidays, is a perfect time to diet. My own opinion is that eating correctly should not be a seasonal matter. *Now* is as good as any time. So start today—not tomorrow!

general hints about good eating habits

1. Meals should definitely not be monotonous. Use your ingenuity. It is important that food be attractive looking, and there should be contrasts in texture, flavor, and color.

2. Try to eat in pleasant surroundings and with enjoyable tablemates. Soft music and soft lights should accompany meals, not noise or bickering.

3. Sprinkle salt sparingly only. Use a non-caloric sweetener, if you must use any, and drink plenty of water *between* meals.

4. If you are reducing, give a lift to plain dishes with low-caloric garnishes such as mushrooms, herbs, wine vinegar, or lemon juice.

5. "Nibble foods" such as carrots, celery, and other vegetables are friends-in-need to the dieter. They are a good way for you to be kind to yourself when you feel hungry.

6. Fruits and vegetables lose their vitamins if mishandled. For best results, cook them as soon as possible after picking or buying. Never cut them too far in advance before a meal, and don't soak them in water. Don't add bicarbonate of soda to the cooking water, as it destroys vitamins B_1 and C. If vegetables are to be stored, store them raw in a cool, but not icy, place.

7. Though I never recommend carrying a calorie-counting book, it may be handy to have one at home to consult occasionally, particularly in relation to alcoholic drinks. Fancy mixed drinks are much more fattening than those made with plain water or soda. Another problem for the dieter is that liquor stimulates the appetite and offers the temptation to forego solid, essential foods. The trimmings such as olives, cheese, and crackers are, of course, all highly caloric. Consistent consumption of liquor also causes trouble of other sorts: it is bad for the

tissues of the skin and tiny nerve endings. But if you can't eliminate alcohol altogether, at least cut down on it.

8. Never eat when you are overtired or upset. This is bad for the digestion, and particularly applies to those who are trying to gain weight. Make an effort to relax first, as tension can undo all the benefits of a well-balanced meal and carefully counted calories.

9. Whether you want to lose or not, do not skip meals, particularly breakfast. Morning calories are more efficiently utilized for energy than those you consume at dinner, when all you have to use them for is sleep.

10. Never sink into an easy chair or take a nap directly after meals. Move about lightly, not vigorously. A short walk is ideal.

11. Never forget or underestimate the role Body Rhythms play in burning calories, as well as toning and firming muscles.

From now on, it should be easy for you to hold on to your determination to succeed in retraining your eating habits. You will find that eating carefully regulated meals, imaginatively planned for their health-giving benefits, will be a stimulating and pleasurable experience.

the dangers of
dehydration

The controversies that center on the use of water are almost unending. Should water be taken during meals? Should you drink water while trying to reduce? Should more water be consumed in the summer, less in the winter? These questions are all easily answered when you understand the part water plays in the human body.

About 70 percent of the body's weight is made up of water. Daily, however, the body gives off about four and one-half pints of its water content. This takes place as follows: about one-half of this amount, consisting of urea, uric acid, and other waste matter from the breakdown of proteins, is excreted through the kidneys. A little more than a quarter is eliminated by the skin through the pores as sweat and sebaceous matter containing some fats. A little less than a quarter is eliminated by the lungs in the form of a watery vapor, which consists of waste matter from the breakdown of carbohydrates and fats. About 2 percent of the water content escapes through the bowels.

So that our bodies can function normally, this large amount of fluid must be replaced. Since the body manufactures less than half the amount of fluid it excretes, the balance must be supplied by the daily intake of food and fluids. This means that nearly two and a half pints must be taken in daily in actual liquid form. A considerable portion of this may be consumed in the forms of tea, coffee, soups, or fruit juices. It is advisable, however, that the major portion of this necessary fluid be taken as pure water.

Water is the basic element of life. It is the solution in which we are conceived, and in which we grow in the womb. Water constitutes 85 percent of the gray matter of the brain, more than 90 percent of blood plasma, and 98 percent of saliva content. Water is essential in the regulation of body temperature. It lubricates the internal organs of the body and prevents the slipping of the intestinal coils, as well as the slipping of joint surfaces. These abnormalities may cause discomfort and even pain.

When we go on a strict, low-calorie diet, we lose fat and protein content from our tissues, but can go on living in spite of it. But a loss of only 10 percent of the water content in the body can present a serious problem. A significant water loss has a serious effect on the chemistry of the blood, and a 20 or 22 percent loss can, and often does, result in death.

This is why artificial dehydration, so often used in weight-reduction programs through such mechanical means as sweat boxes, sauna baths, and dehydration pills, is deplorable. When great amounts of fluids are lost due to excessive dehydration, the result is unsightly flabbiness of muscle tissue. The sudden and extreme loss of water will also dry the skin, causing premature lines, particularly in the face. The deprivation of fluids takes its toll in a variety of other ways. Aside from ruining a person's outward appearance, there is a general feeling of depletion and lack of energy.

To counteract these ill effects, improvement of muscle tone is necessary. The only way this can be achieved is through a planned program of physical activities. A loss in weight without daily physical activity is detrimental, and can be irreparable in extreme cases. Only recently has the relationship between normal water content and a fresh, young-looking skin been recognized. It is for this reason that so many new moisturizing skin creams have appeared on the market, claiming to restore youthful freshness to dry skin.

I would like to relate one example of how damaging artificial dehydration can be. Some time ago a new client came to my office and instead of sitting down at my desk she collapsed into the chair, as if she couldn't stand on her feet another second. When I asked her what was wrong, she said, "I am so tired I feel as if I am going to die." She was a fairly young woman, in her thirties perhaps, certainly too young to reach the point of complete physical exhaustion. On further questioning, I found she had been taking dehydrating pills for six or seven years, not only to control her weight but also to keep her hands and feet from constant swelling. To say I was shocked is an understatement. I agreed to help her on one condition: She must immediately stop taking these pills. She gave me her word of honor she would, and evidently did, judging by the amazing transformation that took place in a comparatively short time.

It was heartening to watch her regain stamina and vitality along with reshaping her figure to graceful, normal proportions just by following my program: by practicing Body Rhythms, by following a corrective diet, and by learning how to relax. She is forever grateful and today continues to tell her friends that I practically saved her life.

If you have any further doubt as to the damaging effects of dehydration, just take a look at the plant you have forgotten to water for a while and you will see with your own eyes what could happen to you. First the leaves droop, then the plant loses its luster, and soon all life is gone. The process of deterioration due to lack of moisture is swift, and the changes are devastating. Remember this the next time you decide to lose weight through the process of dehydration.

Pure water does not add weight, because pure water has no calories and is not retained in the muscle tissue. Water, in fact, is the best solvent known. It is assimilated quickly, aiding elimination, circulation, and digestion. That is why a reducing diet high in protein content is most effective in conjunction with several glasses of water a day. Water should not be taken with meals, however, for it will interfere with proper assimilation and digestion by liquefying the food too rapidly. Drink water, then, not with your meals, but on rising, between meals, and before retiring.

Nature has provided the human body with pores, or tiny openings, whose purpose is to regulate the temperature in your body. When your body is overheated the pores open up and help you cool off by sweating. When the body is cold, as in winter, the pores close up to retain the heat in the body. They therefore serve as regulators of body temperature.

By all means increase the intake of water during warm weather. The hotter the day, the more you perspire. The more water you lose through excessive perspiration, the more you need to replenish in order to maintain the proper water balance in the body.

Remember, WATER—just plain, pure water—is the fluid of life, just as bread is the staff of life. A toast to you, then—with water! Take the "water way" to glowing good health, youthful vitality, and long-lasting beauty.

ideal weight?
your luck may not
last forever

Are you one of the lucky ones whose weight is normal and who has no problem keeping it that way? If you are, you are among the very fortunate. Your body's natural metabolic equilibrium is in complete balance, and your hunger for food is only a normal appetite. You probably enjoy eating but do not stuff yourself. Consciously or not, you've hit on the right system of eating just the right amount and the right combination of nourishing foods.

Unfortunately, all good things come to an end eventually. And that includes your ideal weight. Without an increasing, conscious effort to stay in condition as you grow older, problems will arise. So why not start today to prevent those problems? Ideal figure lines cannot last long if your diet is the least bit deficient, if your muscles are not put to proper use, or if nervous tension takes over.

Take a closer look at your personal habits. In a way, women with ideal weight have an even harder problem than either over- or underweights. Because pounds present no problem, you have probably been paying little attention either to the kind of food you eat, or to whether you eat on a well-balanced, nutritionally satisfying schedule. As for your personal habits, while they may not at present be open to any reproach, you may be laying the groundwork for your own decline, and in time, destroying your youthful appearance.

The kind of thing we're talking about is nibbling. The nibbling need is different from the sensation you usually think of as hunger. It can come as the result of having given your stomach the proper quantity of food but not the proper quality! Without the right kind of food to give you energy and strength, your body, sooner or later, will experience a more serious type of craving when tissues, cells, and organs come to lack proper nourishment. This is what nutrition experts call "hidden hunger," but it doesn't stay hidden for long. Some of its symptoms are a pale complexion, lifeless hair, rough skin, poor teeth, and dull eyesight. A general rundown feeling prevails, complete with worry and tension symptoms.

Even if you've given your body the proper nutritional elements it seems to need, you may often still feel hungry—perhaps because you're tired or nervous. But this is no excuse for eating junk food; fresh fruit is always a much wiser and more satisfying choice. If you feel like having a beverage, remember that lemonade, orange juice, or any other fresh fruit drink provides just as much "pick-up," and with countless more nutritional positives than soft drinks, which are loaded with calories and are a bad habit to fall into. And if you must indulge on occasion in alcoholic drinks, remember that the fancier the drink, the more damaging it may be. A drink taken with plain water is the least harmful, from a digestive viewpoint.

But in the main, remember that your best bets always are the reliable basic foods outlined in the section on nutrition. At the end of this section are special diets which should make your meals adequate from the standpoint of complete appetite satisfaction, as well as that of nourishment. If you should begin to experience signs of being rundown, even on a balanced diet, increase your intake of skim milk and be more generous in your servings of meat, fish, poultry, vegetables, and fruit. And add an extra egg or another tablespoon of butter to your breakfast.

You should also practice Body Rhythms on a regular daily basis. Body Rhythms are not only a perfect means of weight control, they also awaken the full strength, flexibility, and beauty of your body. Changing from the casual way of eating you've been used to, to a consciously well-balanced schedule of nutrition and exercise, you will soon begin to see amazing results. Remember: You are lucky you have no undue weight problems, and that you have been able to achieve an equilibrium which keeps you at the constant, normal level. Appreciate your good fortune and strive to keep yourself alive, alert, and able to work, play, and relax.

136

manya kahn 10-day maintenance diet

general diet rules

The 10-Day Maintenance diet is a quality diet, without calorie counting. If at the end of the first week there is a variance in weight—either loss or gain—increase or decrease the quantity, but retain the same variety of food.

1 Butter vegetables moderately.
2 Eat salad with dressings.
3 Drink coffee and tea in your favorite way. If sweetening is desired, use brown sugar or honey.
4 Avoid liquor, all carbonated drinks, spicy foods, and condiments.
5 Drink plenty of water between meals.

Some days you may want to substitute one of the following delicious and healthy liquid fruit combinations for the regular diet lunch. If not at home during lunch hour, put contents in a thermos bottle and take with you.

½ banana, 8 oz. skimmed milk, 4 oz. fresh orange juice. Mix and chill.

6 fresh apricots, 4 oz. fresh skimmed milk, one egg. Mix and chill.

¼ of ripe cantaloupe, 4 oz. skimmed milk, 4 oz. pineapple juice, preferably fresh. Mix and chill.

3 fresh skinned peaches, 2 egg yolks, 4 oz. fresh orange juice. Mix and chill.

1 ripe skinned apple, 1 egg yolk, 4 oz. skimmed milk. Mix and chill.

Liquid diet drinks should be thoroughly mixed in a blender and chilled.

first day

Breakfast
6 oz. fresh orange juice
1 egg, soft-boiled or coddled
1 slice dark bread, toasted, with 1 pat butter
  coffee with 1 tbs. light cream and 1 tsp. brown sugar

Lunch
2 cups fresh vegetable salad with 1 tbs. French dressing
1 slice dark bread with butter
1 baked apple with honey
8 oz. milk or buttermilk

Dinner
6 oz. tomato juice
¼ broiled chicken
2 cooked green vegetables: ½ cup string beans; ½ cup broccoli, with 1 pat butter each
1 cup mixed green salad with French dressing
1 serving prune whip
  tea with lemon

second day

Breakfast
6 oz. fresh grapefruit juice
1 egg, soft-boiled or coddled
2 pieces Melba toast with 1 pat butter
1 cup coffee with light cream and brown sugar

Lunch
  Cooked vegetable plate: ½ cup string beans; ½ cup cauliflower; ½ cup beets; ½ cup spinach
1 baked potato, med.-sized, with 1 pat butter
1 serving stewed, mixed fruit
8 oz. milk

Dinner
6 oz. fruit juice
6 oz. broiled lean steak
1 cup mixed salad (parsnips, string beans) with 1 tbs. French dressing
1 serving fruit pudding
  tea or coffee

third day

Breakfast
6 oz. fresh orange juice
1 egg, soft-boiled or coddled
1 whole wheat muffin with 1 pat butter
  coffee with light cream and brown sugar

Lunch
2 cups fresh fruit salad with cottage cheese and fruit dressing
1 slice dark bread, toasted and buttered
8 oz. milk or buttermilk

Dinner
½ grapefruit
6 oz. broiled halibut or salmon
1 cup cooked spinach
1 baked potato
1 serving fresh, stewed fruit
  tea with lemon

fourth day

Breakfast
6 oz. prune juice
1 scrambled egg (scramble in double boiler with 3 tbs. milk)
2 bread sticks and butter
  coffee with light cream and brown sugar

Lunch
2 3-oz. broiled hamburger patties
1 cup fresh green salad with 1 tbs. French dressing
  rye Melba toast with cottage cheese
  coffee or tea

Dinner
1 serving fresh fruit cup
6 oz. broiled calves' liver
1 cup cooked beets
1 cup cooked peas
1 cup mixed green salad with French dressing
1 piece sponge cake
  tea with lemon

fifth day

Breakfast
½ grapefruit
1 poached egg
1 slice whole wheat bread, toasted, with butter
  coffee with milk and brown sugar

Lunch
6 oz. broiled mackerel or flounder
1 cup cabbage and carrot salad with French dressing
  bread and butter
2 med. slices pineapple
  tea with lemon

Dinner
  6 oz. sauerkraut juice
  6 oz. roast lamb
1½ cups cooked carrots and peas
  1 cup fresh green salad with dressing
  1 slice fruit pie (whole wheat crust)
    tea with lemon

sixth day

Breakfast
6 oz. fresh orange juice
1 scrambled egg
1 blueberry wheat muffin with honey
  coffee with light cream and brown sugar

Lunch
  1 cup cottage cheese
1½ cups pineapple and grapefruit salad with fruit
    dressing
    rye Melba toast and butter
  8 oz. milk or buttermilk

Dinner
1 serving fresh fruit cocktail
6 oz. roast beef
1 cup cooked spinach
1 cup cooked asparagus
1 serving applesauce
  tea with lemon

seventh day

Breakfast
6 oz. fresh orange or grapefruit juice
1 scrambled egg
1 wheat or fruit muffin with honey
  coffee with milk and brown sugar

Lunch
2 cups fresh fruit salad with fruit dressing
  Melba, whole wheat, or rye toast with butter
1 slice lemon cake
8 oz. milk or buttermilk

Dinner
6 oz. tomato juice
6 oz. roast turkey
1 baked sweet potato
1 cup cooked broccoli
1 cup fresh green salad with dressing
1 serving fruit Jell-O
  tea with lemon

eighth day

Breakfast
6 oz. fresh orange juice
1 egg, soft-boiled or coddled
1 slice whole wheat bread, toasted, with butter
  coffee with cream and brown sugar

Lunch
2 cups fresh vegetable salad with French dressing
1 slice dark bread with butter
1 baked apple with honey
8 oz. milk or buttermilk

Dinner
6 oz. tomato juice
¼ broiled chicken
2 cups green vegetables:
    1 cup string beans
    1 cup broccoli
1 serving prune whip
  tea with lemon

ninth day

Breakfast
6 oz. fresh orange juice
1 egg, soft-boiled or coddled
1 whole wheat muffin with butter
  coffee with light cream and brown sugar

Lunch
2 cups fresh fruit salad with cottage cheese and
    fruit dressing
1 slice dark bread, toasted, with butter
8 oz. milk or buttermilk

Dinner
½ grapefruit
6 oz. broiled halibut or salmon
1 cup cooked spinach
1 baked potato, med.-sized
1 serving fresh, stewed fruit
  tea with lemon

tenth day

Breakfast
½ grapefruit
1 poached egg
1 slice whole wheat bread, toasted, with butter
  coffee with milk and brown sugar

Lunch
6 oz. broiled mackerel or flounder
1 cup cabbage and carrot salad with French dressing
  bread and butter
2 med. slices pineapple
  tea with lemon

Dinner
  6 oz. sauerkraut juice
  6 oz. roast lamb
1½ cups cooked carrots and peas
  1 cup fresh green salad with dressing
  1 slice fruit pie (whole wheat crust)
    tea with lemon

whoever said it's pleasing to be plump?

If you are too heavy but haven't been giving your weight too much thought, start doing some hard thinking. Excess pounds not only make you unattractive and less desirable, they may shorten your life as well. That's right: Obesity is not just a cosmetic problem; it is a functional problem as well. As few as five or ten pounds more than your normal weight will tax your heart, kidneys, and every other vital organ, as well as your general well-being. It's not just your beauty that is at stake when you're overweight—it's your life.

For a woman with a full schedule of business or social activities losing weight is not easy. Wherever you go, whatever you do, there's an abundance of fattening food and drink available to you. You'll find it at luncheons, afternoon club affairs, cocktail parties, and fancy dinners. To be able to resist the constant offerings of delicacies, a person has to be blessed with either a birdlike appetite or fantastic willpower. If you are like most of us, you have neither. Therefore, the answer lies in *learning* to resist these temptations until resisting becomes a conscious daily habit, like combing your hair or brushing your teeth.

Instead of resisting temptation, most overweight women resist admitting they have a problem, and resist doing anything about it. One of the most popular excuses for overweight is glandular dysfunction. Medical science, however, is of the opinion that far fewer cases of overweight are glandular than was formerly believed. Then there are those who believe that obesity runs in their families, and that they are just fated to be fat. More often than not, the only things that run in these families are bad eating habits and rampant ignorance about nutrition.

Usually, overweight is due to a combination of two things: too much eating and too little activity. But obesity can also be an emotional problem. For so many of us, sweets were used when we were children to soothe hurt feelings or wounded knees, or as a reward for being good. That's why when you are anxious or unhappy, you reach for foods that give deep satisfaction. These "goodies" are hard to give up. Since you associate food with solace, reward, and happiness, you probably overeat because you may be feeling restless, or perhaps are going through a difficult time in your life.

Whatever the cause, sublimation or temporary relief is too often sought in the tidbit, the snack, the constant little nibble. The woman at home finds ever-present temptation in her all-too-near refrigerator. And overweight women, whether at home or in a restaurant, too often finish off meals with rich desserts. Many freely admit to this form of self-indulgence, and they often apologize it away with: "I know I shouldn't, but. . . ."

This kind of excuse is as old as the sweet tooth itself. Women who overindulge in the wrong foods and do not eat nourishing, well-balanced meals, commonly suffer from "hidden hunger." Although their bodies are really craving sufficient vitamins and minerals, they try to satisfy these hunger pangs by consuming extra sweets and carbohydrates. Is it any wonder that they accumulate more fatty tissue and added poundage?

To compound the problems of poor eating habits, most Americans lack sufficient physical activity in their daily schedules. We choose to ride rather than walk. Our occupations—as executive, professional, clerk, or even homemaker—require only a limited use of a very few muscles, and modern labor-saving devices tend to reduce our range of physical movements even more. The inevitable results are a gradual slowdown and deterioration of the body's normal functions, and a sluggish level of circulation. Under these circumstances, overweight is practically unavoidable.

Accumulation of fat on the female body follows a certain pattern. It collects mostly in areas that are not sufficiently exercised, like the shoulders, diaphragm, abdomen, hips, and thighs. Excess fat at these points tends to pad the body, creating havoc with movement, crowding internal organs too closely, and even throwing them out of line. Posture, too, is severely impaired by excessive weight. Normal breathing and circulation are thrown off, and motion becomes slow, difficult, and clumsy. Weight adds years to appearance, restricting the clothes a person can wear, and the fun she can have. Even a bright outlook on life may be dimmed. If this is all happening to *you,* the only solution is to do something about your problem, and *do it now!*

The first order of business is to get a medical check-up. You may just be that rare person whose overweight is really caused by an organic disturbance. Only a doctor can tell you whether you are physically fit to go ahead and correct your obesity sensibly and safely.

From then on—it's all up to you! Decide on some nice, selfish, egotistical reason why you want to have a better figure—for that exciting and important weekend, for that beautiful slim, black, size ten evening dress, for that terrific new man, or for getting some romance back into your marriage. Make the reason important enough to outweigh all the other daily motives that make you eat excessively. Make it meaningful enough to keep out of that refrigerator or cookie jar.

beware of temporary measures

There are many, many methods of reducing you can choose from. Unfortunately, most are faddish, illusory, temporary, or even dangerous in their effects. Too frequently, in the hope of achieving quick results, women resort to so-called quick-and-easy methods: starvation diets, reducing pills, cathartics and purgatives, artificial and excessive dehydration, and a variety of mechanical contraptions. I have discussed the crash diet previously; now a word about the others.

Reducing pills This kind of tampering with the body's highly sensitive metabolic system can result in unwanted and often serious side effects. Only in rare instances do such means prove necessary or beneficial. Unless prescribed by your personal physician who can carefully watch over you, they are to be completely avoided.

Cathartics and purgatives These so-called remedies tend to rush food through the digestive system before it has had a chance to be assimilated; the body, therefore, is robbed of its proper nutrients. It weakens and health declines. You might just as well stop eating altogether. This is one of the most unnatural and harmful ways to try to lose weight.

Steam baths and saunas Women have been using steam baths and saunas for years in the belief that perspiration artificially induced by excessive heat will break up fatty tissue. Nothing could be further from the truth! What artificially induced heat does succeed in doing is drawing vital, youth-giving fluids out of the muscle tissues. The body may be left a pound or two lighter, but it is also left lacking in muscle tone. Artificial dehydration puts a strain on the heart, the blood pressure, and on other vital organs. And that isn't all the harm it does.

As we grow older, our bodies—due to metabolic and glandular changes—lose the ability to retain all the necessary fluids in tissues to keep the skin young and firm. Skin begins to dry and sag. Using dehydrating devices such as steam baths and saunas merely helps the aging process along, especially on the face, neck, and skin! Once a woman becomes aware of these important truths, she is bound to reject such drastic measures in any weight reduction program. (And see section on the dangers of artificial dehydration.)

Vibrating tables et al. Several fortunes have been made in promoting mechanical contraptions for weight control, such as rowing machines, vibrating tables, rotating straps, mechanical massagers, and many others too numerous to mention. With most of these mechanical aids, all you lose is time, energy, and money, sometimes a great deal of all three. Nature never intended a human being to rely on these artificial means to preserve good health and good looks. Instead of shaping the muscle structure to graceful, feminine, slender lines, these contraptions encourage unsightly bulges and harden both fatty and muscle tissues. Bulging muscles look good on men; the same can hardly be said for women!

The last resort Tight girdles, often the last resort for a figure gone wild, may give the large body a neater look, but they

140

also encourage the flabby, inert muscles of the diaphragm, abdomen, hips, and thighs to almost cease their natural functioning. Tight girdles are nothing but a prop for lazy muscles to lean on. The best thing you can do for a neater appearance until you slim down is to wear light, resilient two-way stretch garments. Besides giving your body a smoother, better groomed look, they will not crowd or cramp internal organs into unnatural positions. And they won't give your figure that solid, hard, unyielding look.

After all these discouraging facts, here's good news for you.

you can lose weight easily, safely, naturally

To reduce properly, you must decrease your intake of food, particularly carbohydrates and fats, and increase your output of energy. It's as simple as that!

A healthful reducing diet should consist mainly of proteins—meat, fowl, fish, cheese, eggs and milk. Mineral- and vitamin-supplying foods, fresh vegetables and ripe fruits, are also important. What you must not eat, of course, are gravies, cream desserts, and rich dressings. Eat whole grain foods in moderation. When you reduce your consumption of sugars and starches, your body will begin to utilize your own stored-up fat for its daily energy requirements. The fatty tissue will literally begin to break up into fluids, which can then be gradually eliminated through various organs of the body. A well-balanced diet provides all the nourishment and energy your body needs while the surplus fatty tissue is being eliminated. A smaller amount of well chosen, well-balanced food items, rich in proteins, vitamins, and minerals, gives far more nourishment and satisfaction than a diet bulky with fats, sugars, and starches.

As a rule, the first few days of dieting are the toughest. You may feel peevish, hungry, and tired because your stomach has been accustomed to a much larger quantity of food and, of course, it's going to complain at first. Just grin and bear this initial stage. In a few days your stomach will shrink, and the going will be easier.

After a few weeks of shedding pounds and inches, you may suddenly find that you have stopped losing weight, even though you have been following your diet to the letter. This is the curious "dieter's plateau" that comes about when fluids stored in the body tissues replace the fat you have burned up. Psychologically, this is the most dangerous period in dieting because you'll be tempted to stop. Don't! In a little while, if you stick to your diet, you will start losing again.

Working women may have a special problem with dieting. Few restaurants serve foods without sauces and gravies. If you work, you may want to pack your own lunch or find a good cafeteria that has a greater choice of unadorned but wholesome dishes.

A well-proportioned figure is the secret of health, grace, and beauty, and dieting alone cannot achieve it. Exercise and relaxation, of course, go hand in hand with improved diet. You must be active and energetic to help burn off the surplus fat stored in the body. Besides the exhilarating daily Body Rhythms routine outlined for you in this book, you should also practice outdoor activities like tennis, golf, and swimming whenever possible.

Relaxation helps you digest and assimilate food properly, and it can help induce the peace of mind and optimistic attitude you really need for a successful weight reduction program. Try to eat when you are relaxed and not tired. If you are tired, take a short rest period before eating.

Correct breathing is an important adjunct to a successful diet. Each full, deep breath you take flushes the body with oxygen, activates the breathing muscles, and encourages the burning of stored, excess fatty tissue. Try taking long walks, breathing deeply and rhythmically. Carry yourself as tall and as straight as you can. This will stretch your muscles, and it will also make you look thinner.

In conclusion, let me assure you that by following my program for weight loss as described in this section, you will succeed in taking years off your face, lose the extra pounds and inches off your figure, and reshape your body to graceful feminine proportions.

Furthermore, by taking a good look at yourself in the mirror after only a short time, you will discover a more spirited, more attractive, lovelier you!

manya kahn 10-day weight-loss diet

general diet rules

1 Breads permitted on this diet are rye, whole wheat, pumpernickel, rye Melba toast, whole wheat, bran, or corn muffins. Preferably toasted. Any bread on the diet list may be substituted for those suggested in menus.

2 Butter: one small pat ¼-inch thick is allowed for each meal.

3 Coffee and **Tea** is limited to two cups a day without sugar. Demitasse on the meals are bonuses.

4 Dressings on salads should consist of lemon juice with vegetable oil only (1 tablespoon of each) and may be seasoned with a little pepper and salt with garlic if desired.

5 Fish should be broiled with a small amount of vegetable oil and lemon juice.

6 Fruit juices may be fresh, frozen, or canned and should be unsweetened.

7 Meats and **fowl** should be trimmed of all fat before broiling. Meats are broiled with nothing added, except liver which is broiled with a very small amount of vegetable oil. Specified weights are for boneless meat.

8 Salt and pepper can be used in moderation.

9 Snacks of raw celery or carrots are permitted if you are hungry between meals.

10 Vegetables should be cooked in the least possible amount of water and seasoned with salt, pepper and lemon juice only. You may also flavor them with a little fat-free natural gravy from the meat.

11 Water should be drunk between meals only. Drink at least 4 glasses daily, but preferably 6 or 8 glasses.

See also formulas for Liquid Diet Lunches on page 137.

first day

Breakfast
4 oz. fresh orange juice
1 scrambled egg (scramble in a double boiler with 3 tbs. milk)
  Melba toast
  black coffee

Lunch
Fresh fruit cup mixed with cottage cheese
Melba toast
black coffee or tea with lemon

Dinner
6 oz. tomato juice
6 oz. broiled lean steak
1 cup cooked string beans
2 pieces rye Melba toast
  segments of ½ grapefruit or 1 sliced orange

second day

Breakfast
4 oz. orange or grapefruit juice
1 scrambled egg
1 slice rye toast
  black coffee

Lunch
6 oz. tomato juice
6 oz. broiled filet of sole or flounder
½ cup cole slaw with 1 tbs. vegetable oil, plus 1 tbs. lemon juice
1 slice whole wheat toast
  tea with lemon

Dinner
6 oz. orange or grapefruit juice
½ small broiled chicken
1 cup cooked carrots
  sliced lettuce & tomato
2 pieces rye Melba toast
1 baked apple with 1 tsp. honey mixed with 1 tsp. lemon juice
  demitasse

third day

Breakfast
½ grapefruit
3 oz. broiled ham
1 slice pumpernickel bread
  black coffee

Lunch
1 hard-boiled egg
  sliced cucumber, celery, radishes with 1 tbs. vinegar or lemon juice, or vinegar mixed with 1 tbs. vegetable oil
2 pieces rye Melba toast
8 oz. skimmed milk or buttermilk

Dinner
6 oz. tomato juice
6 oz. broiled lean hamburger steak
1 cup stewed celery and tomatoes
1 cup canned low-calorie peaches, drained
1 slice rye toast
  tea with lemon

fourth day

Breakfast
1 fresh orange, sliced
1 poached egg
1 slice rye toast
  black coffee

Lunch
6 oz. salmon or swordfish
1 cup cooked cauliflower
1 sliced tomato
2 pieces rye Melba toast
8 oz. plain yogurt

Dinner
6 oz. broiled calves' liver
1 cup boiled white onions
1 small baked potato or potato boiled in jacket
1 serving low-calorie fruit-flavored gelatin dessert
  tea with lemon

fifth day

Breakfast
6 oz. grapefruit juice
1 boiled egg
1 toasted bran muffin
1 cup black coffee

Lunch
Cooked vegetable plate: carrots, spinach, cauliflower, 1 small baked potato or potato boiled in
jacket with 1 tsp. dairy sour cream
8 oz. skimmed milk or buttermilk

Dinner
6 oz. tomato juice
6 oz. broiled fish or lean meat
1 cup cooked spinach
1 cup cooked beets
1 slice pumpernickel bread
1 stewed fresh pear sweetened with 1 tsp. honey
mixed with 1 tsp. lemon juice
demitasse

sixth day

Breakfast
6 oz. orange juice
1 poached egg on 1 slice rye toast
black coffee

Lunch
8 oz. non-creamed cottage cheese with mixed fresh
fruit
2 pieces rye Melba toast
tea with lemon

Dinner
6 oz. tomato juice
½ small broiling chicken stewed with vegetables:
carrots, celery, green pepper, small white onions, parsley
2 pieces rye Melba toast
4 oz. fresh fruit cup
black coffee

seventh day

Breakfast
6 oz. grapefruit juice
2 eggs, boiled or poached
1 toasted corn muffin
black coffee

Lunch
6 oz. lean roast beef or lamb
mixed green salad with 1 tbs. lemon juice or vinegar mixed with 1 tbs. vegetable oil or 1 tbs.
low-calorie dressing
1 toasted muffin
black coffee

Dinner
6 oz. vegetable juice cocktail
8 oz. broiled lean steak
1 cup cooked broccoli
1 cup cooked white onions
2 pieces rye Melba toast
1 stewed fresh pear sweetened with 1 tsp. honey
mixed with 1 tsp. lemon juice
coffee or demitasse

eighth day

Breakfast
juice of ½ grapefruit
1 soft-boiled egg
1 slice wheat toast
black coffee with skimmed milk, if desired

Lunch
4 oz. tomato juice
4 oz. broiled hamburger
1 cup tossed green salad
8 oz. skimmed milk or black coffee

Dinner
1 cup clear bouillon
6 oz. broiled filet of scrod
1 cup boiled spinach
small portion cole slaw with 1 tbs. vegetable oil
and 1 tbs. lemon juice
fresh fruit cup
tea with lemon

ninth day

Breakfast
1 med.-sized orange, sliced
2 oz. broiled sliced ham
1 piece Melba toast
8 oz. skimmed milk or black coffee

Lunch
1 scrambled egg with ½ cup cottage cheese
1 cup cooked asparagus
2 pieces Melba toast
8 oz. skimmed milk or black coffee

Dinner
2 broiled lamb chops
1 small baked potato
1 cup cooked string beans
1 baked apple with 1 tsp. honey and lemon juice

tenth day

Breakfast
½ grapefruit
1 serving ready-to-eat protein cereal
8 oz. skimmed milk, black coffee, or tea with lemon

Lunch
Cooked vegetable plate: asparagus; 1 small baked potato;
1 tomato; 1 hard-boiled egg
8 oz. buttermilk or black coffee

Dinner
4 oz. broiled fresh salmon
1 cup tossed green salad with 1 tbs. diet dressing
1 cup cooked squash
1 piece Melba toast
1 cup low-calorie gelatin

slender is attractive, but skinny is not!

So many oversized women look at someone who is underweight and sigh, "Why couldn't I be that skinny?" Well, if you have an underweight problem, you know only too well that being skinny can be just as upsetting as being plump. Curiously enough, there are twice as many underweight people in the country as there are obese ones. Yet there seems to be much less concern, much less written about this condition, and much less help available. Perhaps more emphasis has been placed on weight reduction because obesity is considered so much more dangerous to health.

Oddly enough, you have a lot in common with your overweight friends in trying to solve your problem. There are three important rules which apply to both. First, you must get a medical check-up. This is especially important if you are underweight. Failure to gain weight may be due to various physical problems, glandular disturbances, possible chronic infections, digestive upsets, tension, or fatigue. The simple inability to relax can keep you thin as a rail, but only your doctor can diagnose and help you correct your particular condition. Second, underweights, too, must get in the habit of eating three square meals a day, meals that are nutritionally correct and well balanced. This calls for a determination not to skip meals. Quick, inadequate snacks at odd intervals will never help you gain weight. Third, a program of physical activities, both outdoors and indoors, is essential.

Underweight is a more difficult problem to solve than overweight, and most weight-gaining programs do not strike at the real root of the problem. The usual prescription urges the underweight to consume great quantities of food, largely starches and sweets, whether the appetite is there or not. A great deal of rest is also generally prescribed.

On the surface, this kind of advice seems fairly reasonable.

It would seem obvious that anyone would increase poundage merely by being overstuffed and by exerting herself as little as possible in order not to burn up calories. But things are not always as they seem—and particularly not for thin people! Underweights usually suffer from a generally rundown condition, sluggish circulation, and poor muscle tone. When vitality is low, the body is not able to digest and assimilate its nourishment properly. Therefore, a regimen to overload the stomach with an improperly balanced diet will only aggravate the existing condition. The advice to rest and to engage in a minimum of physical activity is equally erroneous: inactivity only increases sluggishness and lack of vitality, often resulting in nervous tension and unhappiness.

Now that you know what not to do, what about the things you *should* do to overcome your feeling of lassitude, to increase your feminine curves, and to rejuvenate you physically and mentally? If you are too thin, there is a diet for you that builds muscle tissue and is accompanied by a program of daily physical activities, improved deep breathing, and proper relaxation.

In planning diets for the thin, emphasis must be placed not on gaining *fat* tissue, but on developing *muscle* tissue. The bulk of the diet should consist primarily of a great variety of proteins: meats, fish, fowl, cheese, eggs, and milk—plus all of the protective foods that supply necessary vitamins and minerals, preferably fresh green vegetables and ripe fruits. You should also have whole-grain breads with your meals, like whole wheat, rye, or pumpernickel. The health desserts indicated on the accompanying weight-gaining diet are a must. You may also eat between meals, but only when you are hungry. It might be best for you to set a regular time for in-between snacks. If you do, stick to the time schedule faithfully.

Remember that it isn't how much you eat, but what you eat and how well you digest and assimilate it that is most important.

Aside from eating well, you must also develop good muscle tone, pleasing contours, and correct posture. Body Rhythms will energize and revitalize your entire body almost effortlessly. As these gentle Body Rhythms stretch, contract, and relax your muscles, blood circulation will accelerate and muscular tone will improve. The heightened circulation will then carry nourishment to every part of your body, helping it grow firm and develop into soft feminine curves. While your new diet program is building new tissue, Body Rhythms will shape and distribute the tissue to the areas that need it most. Where only angles previously existed, new firm, round curves will appear. Your new physical activities will also develop your appetite. In fact, don't be surprised if they make you ravenously hungry—a state you probably didn't know you could achieve. You'll be pleased with your new appetite and your new vitality and energy.

Now, it may be that you are an unusually restless, nervous, and tense person, and that even the ideal program of new, wholesome food habits and physical activities seems not to be enough to help you gain weight. Your restlessness may be using up energy faster than food can provide it. If this is true, you are forgetting an important part of the program: how to relax. Even if the cause of your trouble is a continuing emotional dissatisfaction—perhaps with your occupation, home, or social life—learning how to relax can do wonders. It can set off a wonderful chain of events that will put you on the road to better health and its companion, greater happiness.

If you want to get the full benefit of your newly acquired, wholesome eating habits, a sense of serenity and relaxation should precede all your meals. Make it a ritual to lie on your back on a firm surface for ten or fifteen minutes before dinner. In this position, practice a few Body Rhythms. You will be amazed at how quickly this will dissipate tension and fatigue and give you a feeling of rest and relaxation. For better digestion, learn to eat your food more slowly and never force yourself to eat when you are not hungry.

Relaxing before bedtime is another hint for the underweight woman. The importance of good, sound sleep cannot be overemphasized. Sleep is restorative, revitalizing, and one of the necessities of life; we could not live without it. If sleep is postponed for too long, both physical and mental processes start to deteriorate almost immediately, and serious difficulties result. When restful sleep takes over, the cares and worries of the day fade away completely. "Beauty rest" is of maximum importance and makes every other beauty tip inconsequential by comparison.

The number of hours of sleep needed by individuals varies, but it is generally at least eight, and in underweight cases, as much as ten. If you are a reasonably sound sleeper, you should be able to do with fewer hours than can a restless, light sleeper.

Look for more detailed health hints in the section on relaxation. Once you learn how to relax, you will be free of the tired, haggard feeling that comes from accumulated tension. You will find greater enthusiasm for your new way of life. And you will be a far more interesting and attractive person, as well as a more curvaceous one!

145

manya kahn 10-day weight-gain diet

general diet rules

The 10-Day Weight-Gain diet is a quality diet, without calorie counting. If at the end of the first week there is no gain in weight, increase your food intake, but maintain the variety of food. Let your scale be your guide in the quantity of food you require.

1 Eat vegetables with butter.
2 Eat salads with dressings.
3 Drink coffee and tea with cream and sugar, using brown sugar or honey instead of white sugar whenever possible.
4 Avoid alcohol, all carbonated drinks, spicy foods and condiments.
5 Drink plenty of water between meals.

first day

Breakfast
6 oz. fresh orange juice
2 eggs, soft-boiled or poached
2 slices rye toast with butter
    coffee with light cream and brown sugar

Lunch
    Cooked vegetable plate:
    ½ cup beets
    ½ cup string beans
    ½ cup broccoli
1 baked potato, med.-sized, with 1 pat butter
    bread and butter
1 baked apple with honey
8 oz. milk or buttermilk

Dinner
6 oz. tomato juice
8 oz. hamburger steak
1 cup cooked cauliflower
1 cup cooked spinach
1 cup fresh green salad with 1 tbs. French dressing
1 slice prune pie
    coffee with light cream and sugar

second day

Breakfast
6 oz. fresh orange juice
2 eggs, soft-boiled or poached
1 wheat and fruit muffin with honey
    coffee with cream and sugar

Lunch
8 oz. broiled calves' liver
1 cup lettuce and tomato salad with French dressing
1 slice whole wheat or rye toast and butter
1 piece sponge cake
8 oz. milk or buttermilk

Dinner
1 serving fresh fruit cup
8 oz. broiled lean steak
1 cup cooked cauliflower
1 cup cooked beets
1 serving lemon custard
8 oz. milk or buttermilk

third day

Breakfast
6 oz. fresh orange juice
2 eggs, soft-boiled or poached
2 Graham rolls with butter and honey
    coffee with cream and sugar

Lunch
    Cooked vegetable plate:
    ½ cup beets
    ½ cup string beans
    ½ cup broccoli
    ½ cup spinach
1 baked potato, med.-sized, with butter
    bread and butter
1 slice fruit cake
8 oz. milk or buttermilk

Dinner
½ grapefruit with honey
2 4-oz. broiled lamb chops
1 cup cooked spinach
1 cup cooked peas
1 cup fresh green salad with French dressing
2 fresh peach halves
    coffee with cream and sugar

fourth day

Breakfast
6 oz. fresh orange juice
2 eggs, soft-boiled or poached
2 slices whole wheat or rye toast with butter and honey
    coffee with cream and sugar

Lunch
2 cups fresh fruit salad with cottage cheese and fruit dressing
    whole wheat or rye toast and butter
    fruit cookies
8 oz. milk or buttermilk

Dinner
6 oz. fresh grapefruit juice
8 oz. sliced roast beef
1 cup cole slaw
1 cup cooked broccoli
1 cup cooked squash
    bread and butter
1 piece sponge cake with 1 serving applesauce
8 oz. milk or buttermilk

fifth day

Breakfast
8 oz. prune juice
2 eggs, soft-boiled or poached
2 slices dark bread with butter and fruit jelly
   coffee, milk, or buttermilk

Lunch
8 oz. broiled filet of sole
1 cup cooked spinach
1 baked potato, med.-sized
1 cup lettuce and cucumber salad with French
   dressing
   bread and butter
1 serving custard
8 oz. milk

Dinner
1 cup fresh vegetable soup
8 oz. broiled calves' liver
1 cup cooked string beans
1 cup fresh green salad with French dressing
1 serving stewed pears
8 oz. milk

Breakfast
6 oz. fresh orange juice
2 eggs, soft-boiled or poached
2 fruit muffins with butter and honey
   coffee or tea with cream and sugar

sixth day

Lunch
2 cups fresh fruit salad with cottage cheese and
   fruit dressing
   whole wheat or rye toast and butter
1 baked apple
8 oz. milk or buttermilk

Dinner
1 cup fresh vegetable soup
8 oz. broiled lean steak
1 cup mashed potato
1 cup cooked beets
1 cup fresh green salad with French dressing
   bread and butter
1 slice apple pie
   coffee with cream and sugar

seventh day

Breakfast
6 oz. fresh orange juice
2 scrambled eggs
2 fruit muffins with butter and honey
   coffee with cream and sugar

Lunch
1 serving fresh fruit cup
2 4-oz. hamburger patties
1 cup fresh green salad with French dressing
   toast and butter
1 serving ice cream with fresh strawberries
8 oz. milk

Dinner
6 oz. tomato juice
½ broiled chicken
1 cup cooked squash
1 cup cooked broccoli
   bread and butter
1 slice fruit pie
   tea with cream and sugar

eighth day

Breakfast
6 oz. fresh orange juice
2 eggs, soft-boiled or poached
2 Graham rolls with butter and honey
   coffee with cream and sugar

Lunch
2 cups fresh fruit salad with cottage cheese and
   fruit dressing
   whole wheat or rye toast and butter
   fruit cookies
8 oz. milk or buttermilk

Dinner
6 oz. fresh grapefruit juice
8 oz. sliced roast beef
1 cup cooked broccoli
1 cup cooked squash
1 cup cole slaw
   bread and butter
1 piece sponge cake with 1 serving applesauce
8 oz. milk or buttermilk

ninth day

Breakfast
6 oz. fresh orange juice
2 eggs, soft-boiled or poached
2 slices whole wheat or rye toast with butter and
   honey
   coffee with cream and sugar

Lunch
2 cups fresh fruit salad with cottage cheese and
   fruit dressing
   whole wheat or rye toast and butter
   fruit cookies
8 oz. milk or buttermilk

Dinner
½ grapefruit with honey
2 4-oz. broiled lamb chops
1 cup cooked spinach
1 cup cooked peas
1 cup fresh green salad with French dressing
2 fresh peach halves
   coffee with cream and sugar

tenth day

Breakfast
8 oz. prune juice
2 slices French toast with fruit jelly
   coffee with cream and sugar
8 oz. milk or buttermilk

Lunch
8 oz. broiled fish
1 cup cooked spinach
1 baked potato, med.-sized
1 cup lettuce and cucumber salad with French
   dressing
   bread and butter
1 serving custard
8 oz. milk

Dinner
1 cup fresh vegetable soup
8 oz. broiled calves' liver
1 cup cooked string beans
1 cup fresh green salad with French dressing
1 serving stewed pears
8 oz. milk

care of
problem areas

The bosom is our most essentially feminine attribute and it is symbolic of all forms of nurturing. It has been immortalized in all styles and periods of art, and in its broader and more generous use, the word bosom is synonymous with a haven or a refuge, because of its deep association with love, safety, peace, and rest.

Current fashion assumes the bosom to be very adaptable. This is a fortunate state of affairs, because while the flat-chested can always wear padded bras, the woman with a large bosom can be fitted into a bra that minimizes the size and gives it a desirable feminine contour. It is heartening to know that most bosom problems can be solved healthfully and sensibly. The usual problems are breasts that are too large or too underdeveloped, or are flabby and tend to sag. The bosom will respond to the same corrective procedures as the rest of the body—diet, exercise, and good posture. In fact, the bosom is often more adaptable to refashioning than other parts of the body. This is because there are no bones in the breasts, as there are in the hips, for example, where weight may be reduced or added, but where bone structure determines basic size and shape. An understanding of the difference in structure and function of the breasts from the rest of the body will be helpful here.

The breasts function through the mammary glands. These glands are composed of many lobes and lobules, tiny tubes or ducts that carry the mother's milk to the nipple at the time of childbirth.

The nipple, more darkly pigmented than the rest of the body, is a muscular organ with fifteen to twenty tiny pore openings through which the milk is drawn. Because the nipple is muscular, it can become hard and erect through contraction due to cold, excitement, fright, or friction from rough clothing.

The remainder of the breast is largely connective tissue cushioned by a fatty layer. Supporting the breasts are several sets of muscles and ligaments. Some of these reach upward to the collarbone, almost like imaginary lingerie straps. Others fan outward to the chest muscles. It is the health and elasticity of these muscles that affect the shape, size, and firmness of the breasts.

Due to the delicate construction of the breasts, no harsh treatment should ever be given to this part of the body. Massage or mechanical means of reshaping this area are definitely not advised. They tend to hasten the breakdown of tissues, causing a flaccid, sagging condition, rather than strengthening the tissues. They can even cause serious injury.

The proper corrective exercise will strengthen delicate breast muscles to hold the breasts in their proper position, and will develop good posture. Body Rhythms 11–15 are the correct exercises for either developing or minimizing bosom size, and you will be amazed at the wonders these rhythmic movements can work for bosom beauty.

In coordination with exercise, you will need to practice deep, rhythmic breathing, and relaxation, and follow a diet appropriate for your body needs.

While the vogue of today advocates going braless, my own conviction is that a bra, properly fitted, has two important beauty advantages. It gently molds the soft tissues of the breasts into young-looking and fashionable lines. Furthermore, it gives just the right support that the weight of the breasts needs to aid the muscles in holding them high and firm. Unsupported, the breasts, especially if they are large, have a tendency to sag with the years. If you have large bosoms, always exercise wearing a bra.

Your natural bosom structure, like your facial features, is unique! It may not be perfect, but it's yours. And while severe alteration is not practicable—or even desirable—there is a great deal you can do to develop a fine, firm, and lovely bosom line, symmetrical and harmonious to the general lines of your body. It will immeasurably add to your self-confidence as a woman.

lovely hands — the tip-off to good grooming

Your hands are as expressive as your face and as personal as your smile. They are the human instruments of creation, care, and caress. They are continually in the limelight, so why not make them suitable objects of attention? A woman's hands should be beautiful to look at and graceful when in motion.

There was a time when practically all a woman's hands had to do was to wave a fan or twirl a parasol. Then it was easy to have soft, delicate hands. Today, however, we like our hands to look capable as well as feminine—strong but smooth and graceful, with pretty, well-shaped fingernails.

Hands are such useful instruments. They garden, cook, sew, type, play an instrument; but a lot of what they do makes them dirty and rough. Your hands are a complete tip-off to your pride in yourself and your real interest in good grooming habits. It is not enough to give your hands a casual dip in soap and water and consider them well-groomed. You wonder why your hands are rough and chapped? Logically enough, it's because of habits like going gloveless in cold weather, doing dishes in piping hot water, and using your fingernails to pry open jars and untie knots.

protection is essential

These days experts are giving us more and more help on how to keep hands young and smooth, and nails perfectly shaped and shining, despite the destruction wrought by detergents and mechanical devices that seem intent on ripping the nails and coarsening the skin. The skin of the hands is the dryest on the body, because it produces almost no oils of its own, and therefore it ages fastest. The skin needs help, and deserves our special attention.

It is a good idea, in every room in the house where you're apt to wash your hands, to place within easy reach a bar of pure soap, a small handbrush, and a small jar of hand cream or lotion. This means the kitchen, the bathroom, the laundryroom. If you're a working woman, keep handy in your desk drawer a small bottle of lotion and a supply of soft towels. (Most company washrooms supply only paper towels which are bad for your hands.)

Avoid immersing hands in water of extreme temperature, whether too hot or too cold. Whenever you are wearing short sleeves, you should definitely give a thorough going-over to your forearms, elbows, and even upper arms, using brush, soap, and lotion, just as you do your hands. Elbows are dirt-catchers; pay special attention to them. If your hands are stained or discolored, rub a little lemon juice or hydrogen peroxide on the stain, just before you dry them. A pumice stone, gently applied to any rough spots on your fingers, palms, or elbows, will smooth them away in short order.

The next step is protection. When you wash dishes, as well as when you do any housework, light or heavy, wear rubber gloves. Then, there are some useful products provided by modern science. Many lotions, besides softening, moisturizing, and healing, also double as a shield against weather and dirt. Find out which they are and apply them sparingly before tackling any rough or heavy jobs, especially in bitter winter weather. Because our hands are so busy and because we tend to think of their beauty last, they literally get into a lot of difficulties that can spoil their looks, by reddening, roughening, or staining the skin, or by splitting the nails. A simple method of protecting them in advance is to massage cream or lotion into the hands before bedtime and then cover them with an old pair of cotton gloves or a cheap pair purchased for this purpose. You can see in the morning how much cream a pair of thirsty hands can drink up and how refreshed they look after this treatment.

When you are outdoors in cold or windy weather, protect your hands with gloves. Only a few steps without them on a raw day

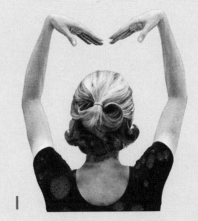
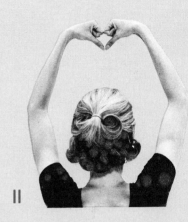

I. Standing with arms relaxed at sides, **breathe in**, raise arms above head, elbows slightly bent. **Breathe out**, stretch hands way down from wrists. Relax hands. **Repeat five times**, breathing in and out.

II. **Breathe in**, clench hands into fists. **Breathe out**, stretching thumbs down. Relax hands. **Repeat five times**.

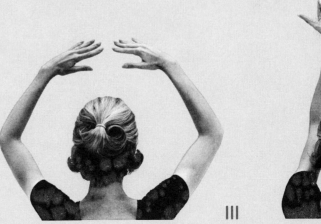
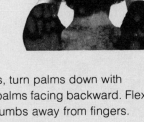

III. Raise arms above head, hands above wrists, turn palms down with thumbs apart. **Breathe in**, stretch arms up with palms facing backward. Flex finger joints tightly and bend into palms with thumbs away from fingers. **Breathe out**. Relax. **Repeat five times**.

IV. Raise arms above head, elbows slightly bent with hands stretched way down from wrists.

Breathe in, clench hands into fists with thumbs stretched up, fists touching.

Breathe out, open hands, stretch fingers up and wide apart. Relax. **Repeat five times.**

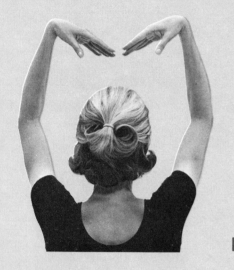

IV

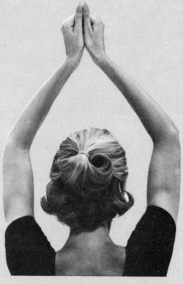

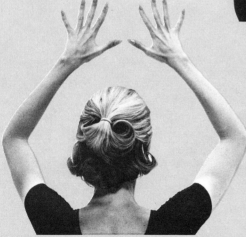

These Body Rhythms will prevent stiffness in the joints and will create flexibility and dexterity. Hands and feet are prone to poor circulation. Practice these movements frequently to correct this difficulty.

can do damage. Indoors, of course, protect your hands against heavy cleaning chores. If you can't wear rubber gloves and your work is going to be particularly dirty, dig your fingernails first into a bar of pure soap. This will prevent dirt from embedding itself there, and will also make cleaning afterward easier. And never, never use your nails on a job that can be done just as well with scissors or pliers.

If, however, in spite of all precautions, one of the following conditions should arise, let me outline the best thing to be done about it.

Chapped hands Keep them covered with hand cream every chance you get. Before bedtime, apply emollient or an extra-rich cream, and sleep with cotton gloves on.

Red hands Use the same suggestions as for chapped hands, and practice the hand exercises in this section. Prop your elbows on a flat surface, holding the hands high until the blood drains down. Do this for about ten minutes at a time at least once a day. Cover the red areas with tinted foundation base until you've eliminated the problem. If redness persists, see your physician, as this redness can be a symptom of one of the various types of eczema that can be treated only under medical supervision.

Weak nails Keep them oiled every chance you get, and be particularly sure to apply cuticle oil at bedtime when your hands are at rest. Use manicure materials with an oily base. White or colorless iodine is a nail strengthener. Apply it a few times a week, especially when your nail polish is off. And *check your diet*. If your fingernails are split, ridged, and breaking, you might take a few moments to check whether your general health is good and your diet correct. Nails take nine months to grow, and the matrix from which they emerge is just below the cuticle. If your basic health was good nine months ago, their general appearance, shape, and quality will be good. Gelatin added daily to fruit juice, milk, or bouillon has been found to be remarkably beneficial for strengthening weak nails. Extra portions of milk and cottage cheese are another good idea, as very brittle nails are caused by lack of calcium.

what about a manicure?

A manicure is not just for beauty. It performs a necessary function by keeping the nails clean, as well as pretty, and is essential to good grooming. If your nails are in poor condition, be careful of your manicuring technique, especially with regard to the cuticle at the nail's base. Work very gently: harsh treatment at this spot—such as bruising from heavy pressure of a cuticle pusher—can cause injury to the soft layers of the nail still being formed. Weak nails should be shaped as closely to the fingertips as is comfortable, for shorter nails will have less tendency to break. Buffing the nails gently is the perfect ending for a manicure, both smoothing the surface and improving circulation to your hands.

You should use *all* the steps of this hand-care routine for best results. Protection and cleanliness, proper exercise, and manicure habits—these will ensure you of the excellent functioning of efficient and lovely hands.

body rhythms aid circulation

Poor circulation can mean clammy, moist palms. If you have this problem, wear a little antiperspirant on the palms. And above all, *exercise.* Hands are subject to circulation problems because they are extremities of the body; this is the reason hands and feet often feel cold. Illustrated here are Body Rhythms designed specifically for circulation problems. The hands should be treated with a rich emollient hand cream before each Body Rhythms session. Make sure the movements of the hand massage are firm and deep, performed by the cushion of the hand and not the fingers only. When applying hand cream after washing and at any other time, apply with correct movements. Rhythm is always important to good, even, effective work. Skill, dexterity, and rhythm above all are ever-present in the efficient, productive work of any pair of hands. Try to develop them through the hand and finger exercises shown here. A light and graceful touch can be fostered by following my instructions carefully. What you do and how you use your hands can add to or detract from your beauty.

general hints for lovely hands

1. Keep hands relaxed; don't fuss with your hair or jewelry. Avoid tense, taut gestures.

2. When standing, your hands should hang naturally at your sides. Avoid placing hands on hips, or clasping them behind your back, which suggests tension and insecurity.

3. When sitting, your hands should rest on your lap, one hand slightly overlapping the other.

4. Never, under any circumstances, clench your hands. Avoid clutching your cards when playing bridge, or when talking to others, as this too is a sign of nervousness and tension.

5. Nail biting I need not even mention. If an appeal to your vanity hasn't been enough to stop this ugly habit, the only thing I can suggest is a consultation with your doctor to help your tension, or to exercise your strongest willpower.

6. Never clean nails with a sharp, metal instrument. You'll risk scraping the nail and damaging its softer portions.

7. Relief for swollen, tired, aching hands can be obtained by soaking them in hot water with a tablespoonful of salt.

8. Avoid, most of all, the limp, lifeless handshake. A firm, strong grip is the warm, friendly and correct outward expression of your inner strength and self-assurance.

healthy feet — the barometer of well-being

The care of feet plays an important and essential part in every health and beauty regimen. Our feet are a very sensitive barometer of our mental and physical state.

Foot discomfort is always mirrored in the face. It can create a painful, suffering expression and even cause lines on the forehead. Most women are smart about the care they give to their bodies, but often seem to draw a blank when it comes to the care of their feet.

Relatively small though they are, feet perform the work of giants. Next to the heart, the feet carry the greatest load of any part of the body. This fact is worth keeping in mind. No other structure could bear such a top-heavy burden for so long and without repairs as the delicate, ingeniously designed human foot. It is a wonder that things go wrong as rarely as they do, considering how poorly feet are understood or cared for.

The foot operates on two flexible arches. The long arch of the instep is known as the longitudinal, and it runs the length of the foot. The arch at the ball of the foot, supporting the width, is the metatarsal. These two arches provide the spring that feet must have to support and balance the weight of the body as we move. Toes and heels help further to balance and move the body effortlessly, but if we had no arches, if the feet were rigid, they would break under the strain of body weight.

Most of the time we are unaware of our feet; this means they are in good working order, strong, and flexible. But even a minor foot problem tends to magnify itself; foot discomfort has a way of spreading to every part of the body. Foot disorders are many, the most common being fallen arches, flat feet, calluses, bunions, and corns. There are a host of others, but their cure is within the realm of medical doctors only. Many troubles can be traced to correctible causes like the following:

Bad posture Poor posture is the prime offender, causing not only weak muscles in the abdomen, hips, and thighs, and rigidity and tension in the spinal column, but extreme strain on legs and feet. It makes proper standing and moving impossible, and must be corrected if foot problems are to be relieved.

Poor circulation Lack of adequate circulation in the feet promotes coldness, dampness, and easy fatigue, as well as making muscles tense and weak. This combination of symptoms can cause walking to be jerky and awkward, so that each step is a shock to the body. Another common effect is swelling, especially around the ankles. The exercises illustrated here are especially designed with the problem of circulation in mind. Bone and muscle structure in ankles, legs, and feet must be strengthened and circulation stimulated. These simple exercises will make your feet feel fresh and young, and make walking a pleasurable pastime.

Overweight Like bad posture, extra pounds throw a tremendous burden on legs and feet. For foot comfort, it is necessary to reduce this excess poundage and create firm, elastic, and strong muscles in areas like the thighs, hips, and abdomen. They will then take their share of body weight from the legs and feet.

Badly fitted shoes Very simply, the size and fit of your shoes must give your feet both ample room and support. High heels, worn more than occasionally, are ruinous to legs and feet. The constant wearing of high heels throws the entire weight of the body onto the metatarsal arch, causing great strain and pressure on an area utterly unequal to the task. High heels also shorten the muscles in the back of the leg and make them rigid. Rather than use them for any kind of lengthy walking, shopping, working, keep your high heels for dressy occasions only. We are lucky today that attractive, low-heeled shoes have been created that are graceful and highly becoming to the feet. Changing heel heights often will rest your feet and keep muscles supple.

All shoes, no matter what their shape or height, ought to meet certain standards of proper fitting. The general rule is that the shoe should be at least half an inch longer than the big toe and should be neither too tight nor too loose. Stand with your full weight on the feet whenever trying on shoes. Each should be roomy at the broadest part of the foot and fit snugly at the heel, under the arch, and over the instep.

treating tired feet

Treatments for plain old tired feet vary. But all are only variations of the basic foot bath, massage, and rest. Plunge your feet into a quart of warm water and add two tablespoons of Epsom salts. Next, immerse them in cold water. Rub with alcohol, then with softening cream. Starting with the toes, massage each one separately, then the ball of the foot, the arch, the heel, and finally the ankle area. Use both hands, placing the palm of one hand on top of the foot and the other underneath. Pressure is applied by the palms, and the strokes should be gentle but firm. Next, prop the feet up—on pillows, on a chair, anywhere, so long as they are higher than your hips. A twenty-minute rest should be sufficient to restore healthy circulation.

The foot bath should be a ritual Proper bathing of the feet, like proper washing of the hands, is a ritual we either never really learned or have forgotten in the hurry of daily life. But you needn't set aside a special session for foot bathing; your daily bath or shower is a perfect occasion for giving them the attention they need.

Like the rest of the body, feet perspire, but because they're usually encased in shoes and stockings, they retain perspiration a great deal more than do less confined areas. Unpleasant odor is the result, as is rough or dead skin, which should be removed before it causes irritation. Foot bathing should be tackled with real vim. Keep a handbrush with moderately stiff bristles nearby and really scrub the feet with it. Use plenty of soap, warm water, and elbow grease, and don't forget the soles! Scrub between the toes with an old toothbrush. Rinse your feet and rub pumice stone, with a gentle rotary motion, over any areas that are partic-

Body Rhythms to stretch and strengthen foot muscles, including the arches of the feet. Practice slowly and thoroughly so that you feel the stretch in the knees, calves, and ankles.

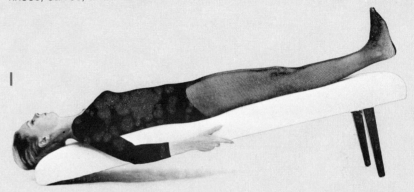

I. With arms at sides, **breathe in**, flex feet toward upper part of body. Stretch heels out, bringing arms up simultaneously. **Breathe out**, point feet and toes out, knees straight. Bring arms to sides. Relax. **Repeat five times.**

With arms at sides, **breathe in** as you flex both feet. **Breathe out** as you point both feet. Alternate movement, flexing and pointing feet as far out as possible. **Repeat five times.**

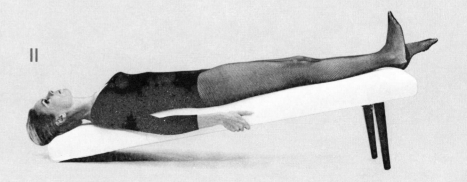

II. **Breathe in**. Point right foot out from ankle and flex left foot inward simultaneously. **Breathe out**. Stretch left foot out from ankle as you flex right foot inward. Alternate movement stretching feet thoroughly with knees straight. **Repeat five times.**

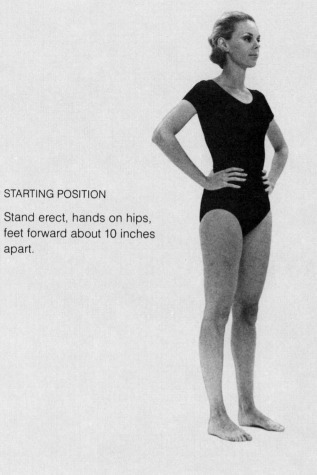

STARTING POSITION

Stand erect, hands on hips, feet forward about 10 inches apart.

III. **Breathe in**, rise on toes with knees straight. **Breathe out**, lower heels to floor. Relax. **Repeat five times.**

III

IV. **Breathe in**, rise on toes, knees straight. **Breathe out**, lower left heel, bending right knee simultaneously. **Breathe in**, rise on toes, lower right heel as you bend left knee. Alternate movements from right to left and left to right. Relax. **Repeat five times.**

IV

V. From Starting Position, **breathe in**, lift inner arch and curl toes under with body resting on outsides of feet. **Breathe out**, relax. **Repeat five times.**

With toes curled and arches lifted, take a few steps forward and then backward. Relax. **Repeat five times.**

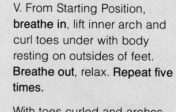

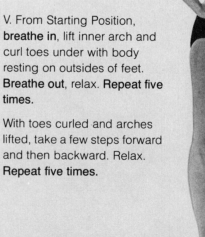

V

156

VI. From Starting Position, **breathe in**, raise both feet upward resting body on heels, knees straight. **Breathe out**, lower feet to floor. Alternate raising and lowering feet, breathing in and out, and keeping knees straight.

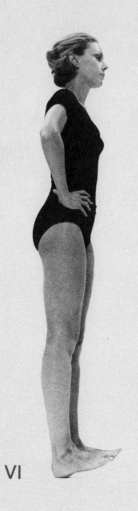

VII. From Starting Position, **breathe in**, raise both feet upward resting body on heels, knees straight. Take a few steps forward and then backward, breathing in and out. Relax. **Repeat five times.**

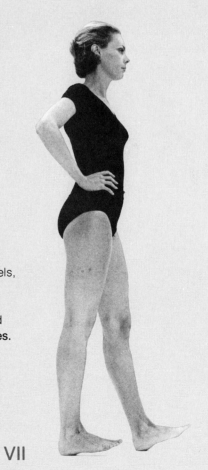

VI

VII

ularly rough. This will soften skin and discourage calluses. Most important is the drying of your feet, which must be absolutely thorough in order to prevent plagues like athlete's foot, a fungus that thrives on warm, damp skin. When you leave your bath, add a quick dab of hand lotion to smooth the rough and chapped spots on your feet, and finish with a dust of talcum powder.

If your feet are plagued by excessive perspiration, massage them with rubbing alcohol just before applying hand lotion. Afterward, substitute an antiseptic powder for plain talcum, as this will have more of a drying effect. Also powder the insides of your shoes for a fresh, cool feeling.

what about a pedicure?

A regular, relaxing pedicure can do wonders for tired feet and, like a new hairdo or facial, can give you a special lift. A good pedicure is as beneficial and beautifying for your feet as a manicure is for your hands, and ought to be done once a week all year round.

First, remove all polish from your toenails. Soak and scrub your feet, dry them, and then apply nail cream to the cuticles. Press back each cuticle gently with a soft cloth. Using a clipper, cut the nails straight across, without curving them down at the edges, and smooth off the cut surfaces with an emery board. Now, separating the toes with balls of cotton, apply a colorless base coat, then a coat of polish. Two coats are necessary because toes come in for much friction, and polish chips quickly. It is a good idea to cover the whole nail in applying polish, as the shape and moons of your toenails are not as well-defined as those of your fingernails. Allow ample time for drying, and apply a coat or two of softening lotion to the feet, massaging them in gently.

general hints for healthy feet

1. To promote foot freedom and muscular development, go barefoot in summer; in winter go barefoot at home wearing socks to keep your feet warm.

2. Make an effort to analyze the way you walk. With feet parallel, about four to six inches apart and toes pointed straight ahead, make a conscious effort to correct either toeing out or in. Keep your weight on the balls and outer edges of the feet.

3. Never wear the same pair of shoes two days in a row, and check your shoes for needed repairs to avoid foot trouble.

4. To avoid constricted circulation in the feet, never wear tight pantyhose.

When you have reached the stage where walking for hours does not fatigue you, you will at last know the meaning of true foot comfort. Walking then will become healthful fun.

a final word about a more feminine, relaxed, lovelier you

By the time you have finished reading this book, you will have acquired a better understanding of your physical self and will realize what it takes to achieve radiant and glowing womanhood. For without a clear picture of what can be achieved it is unlikely that you will have the incentive to strive for good results. All the knowledge in the world will get you nowhere if you don't act. In order to succeed, it is imperative that you take all the necessary steps right now! For there is all the difference in the world between good intentions and deliberate action.

In the days following completion of the 10-Day Program you will become aware of this when your firm resolutions, your hopes and aspirations for a new, more attractive YOU will either fly out of the window or become a reality. Either you will act like the little bird whose life of indolence and pleasure means more to it than ceasing its dissipation, or you will embark on a new and disciplined program needed for success.

Step by step you have learned the seven major principles that will keep you in tip-top form: proper nutrition, good posture, deep breathing, rest and relaxation, the value of fresh air and sunshine. Having read the section on nutrition carefully, you learned that what counts is quality of food and not quantity, and you will never again "fill up" merely to satisfy hunger or a false appetite. By the time you have mastered the valuable techniques of correct posture, deep breathing, and relaxation, you will know that Body Rhythms play a major part in the entire program of self-improvement. This knowledge will encourage you never to pass even one day without exercising, for you will take pride in your newly slimmed, gracefully contoured body. Your new energy will bring new pleasure in outdoor activities. You will have a sense of well-being, and will be happy and glad to be alive.

Finally, I would like to add a few words about our mental and emotional state in relation to health and beauty. The enormous growth in the fields of psychiatry, psychoanalysis, and psychology reveals that there is a close connection between mental and physical health, and points out the need for a plan of living that builds stability of mind and spirit as it builds the body.

During the vibrant years of youth we taste the heady bouquet of acclaim, praise, and admiration. While we thrive on our physical attributes, good looks, and magnetism, we feel certain that life will go on in this rosy state endlessly and happily.

The far-sighted woman, however, looks ahead early in life because she realizes that in time her physical attractions will fade into less prominence, and will have to be replaced by more permanent and lasting qualities.

By the time we reach maturity, with children grown and husbands often absorbed in their careers, many of the interests and activities of our younger years no longer hold our interest and attention. It is at this stage that we begin to lose confidence and self-assurance, causing unnecessary nervousness, self-pity, and mental tension. Now is the time to direct our minds and energies away from home, family, office, and self-absorption. It is at this time that the smart woman develops interests outside her immediate sphere. For the first time she can devote attention to the "outside" world: many women rediscover books and education programs in order to improve their minds and conversation; many develop a keen interest in others.

Life can be infinitely fuller and more meaningful when we devote some of our time to the lives of others, especially the less fortunate ones who need help, love, and compassion. This worthy endeavor—this "giving of ourselves"—brings great satisfaction and fulfillment. This is also a time to develop a constructive hobby and concentrate on it. All in all, the great variety of activities and exciting possibilities within our grasp helps us forget our immediate problems, which, in perspective, can become small and insignificant.

When we reach the dangerous forties and fifties, the first glow of youth begins to dim, the first fine etchings of age show their delicate traces around the eyes and mouth. This is a time to take into account the emotional flurries caused by both physical and mental changes. It is at this period of life that a woman must realize that there is more to life and womanhood than sheer physical beauty. It is only then that the inner qualities begin to develop and express themselves in a calm, serene attitude, healthy thinking habits, a good sense of humor—all of which add up to a mature and healthy outlook on life.

Life can be full of excitement, interest, and fun at any age. And so this book—not just a health and beauty course with a time limit in mind, but a lifelong program to keep you more feminine, more naturally beautiful, and lovelier to look at. And most of all, attractive to know . . . desirable and exciting to be with . . . regardless of age!